The Practical Science-Backed ANTI-INFLAMMATORY DIET COOK BOOK FOR BEGINNERS

Step by Step Plan, 200+ Super Easy Recipes &
A 30-Day Meal Plan to Reset Your Cells, Immunity,
Gut Health And Ease Chronic Pain

ELENA FLORENZ

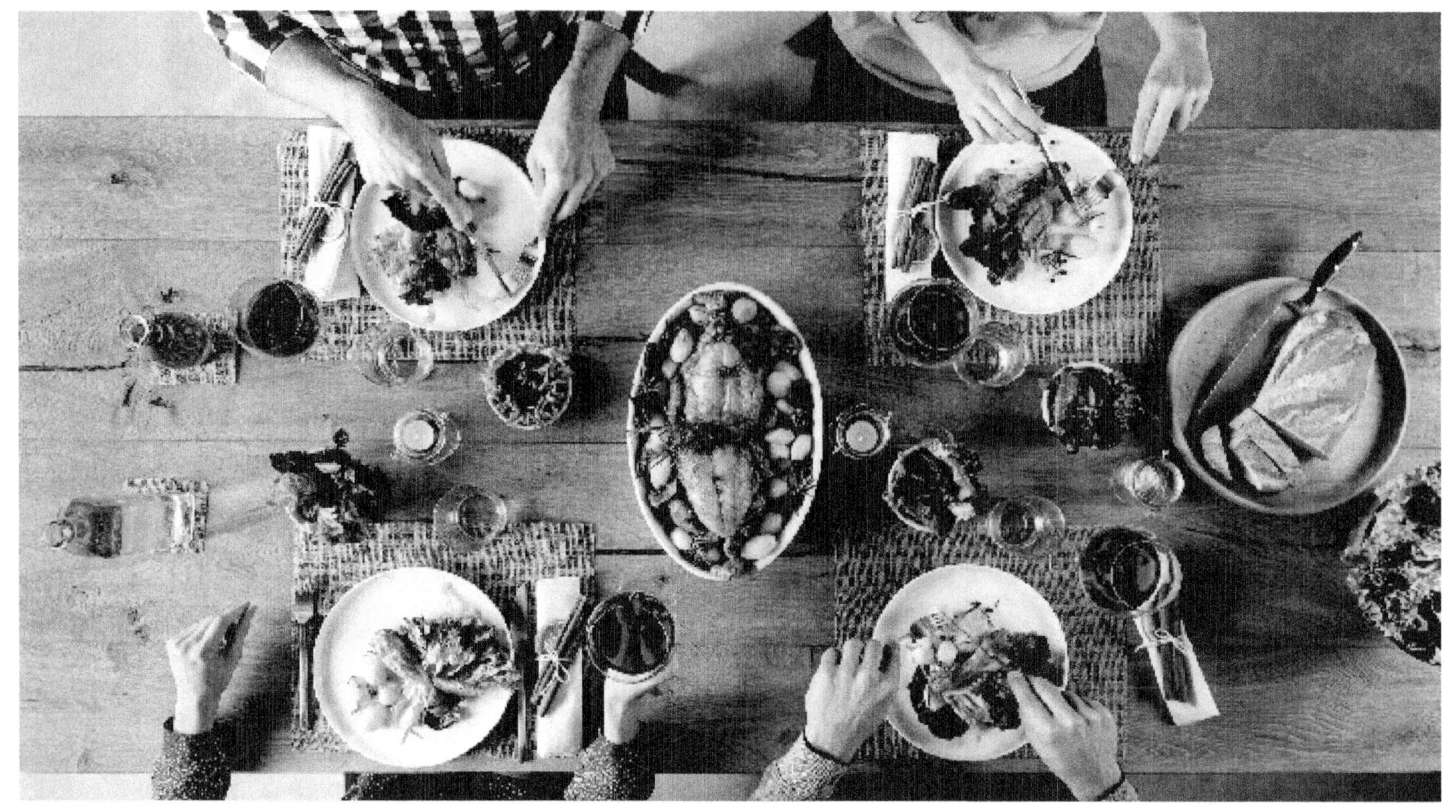

COPYRIGHT © 2024 BEGINNERS

All rights reserved. No part of this book may be reproduced, distributed, or transmitted in any form or by any means, including photocopying, recording, or other electronic or mechanical methods, without the prior written permission of the publisher, except in the case of brief quotations embodied in critical reviews and certain other noncommercial uses permitted by copyright law.

LEGAL NOTICE. The information contained in this book is intended for educational and informational purposes only and is not a substitute for professional medical advice or treatment. Consult with a qualified healthcare professional before making any changes to your diet or lifestyle. The author and publisher expressly disclaim responsibility for any adverse effects that may result from the use or application of the information contained in this book.

DISCLAIMER. While every effort has been made to ensure the accuracy and reliability of the information contained in this book, neither the author nor the publisher can assume responsibility for errors, inaccuracies, or omissions. The reader is advised to consult with healthcare providers for specific health-related issues and should exercise caution when preparing recipes, particularly for allergies and dietary restrictions.

CONTENTS

INTRODUCTION	7
A STEP BY STEP GUIDE: AN OVERVIEW ON HOW TO USE THIS ANTI-INFLAMMATORY DIET COOKBOOK	8
PURPOSE OF THE ANTI-INFLAMMATORY DIET COOKBOOK	9
A PERSONAL JOURNEY FROM PAIN TO EMPOWERMENT THROUGH FOOD	10

CHAPTER 1
ANTI-INFLAMMATORY DIET — 11

CHAPTER 2
GETTING TO KNOW INFLAMMATION — 14

CHAPTER 3
MICROBIOME, IMMUNE SYSTEM AND CELLULAR REGENERATION — 17

CHAPTER 4
EMBRACING AN ANTI-INFLAMMATORY DIET & LIFESTYLE: A PRACTICAL GUIDE — 20

DOWNLOAD YOUR BONUS
ANTI-INFLAMMATORY RECIPE BOOK WITH VIBRANT, FULL COLOR PICTURES — 26

CHAPTER 5
SOUPS AND STEWS — 27

Carrot And Chicken Soup	28
Sweet Potato & Lentil Stew	28
Green Detox Soup	28
Spicy Tomato And Basil Soup	29
Miso And Tofu Soup	29
Quick Broccoli Soup	29
Curried Parsnip And Apple Soup	29
Pumpkin And Corn Soup	30
Okra And Tomato Stew	30
Butternut Squash & Chickpea Soup	30
Quick Anti-Inflammatory Vegetable Broth With Noodles	31
Quick Beef And Potato Stew	31
Moroccan Chicken And Apricot Stew	31
Minestrone Soup	32
Spanish Chorizo And Bean Stew	32
Chickpea And Tomato Stew	32
Zesty Black Bean Soup	33
Turkey And Vegetable Stew	33
Spicy Lemongrass Chicken Soup	33
White Fish Stew	33
Lamb And Eggplant Stew	34
Cauliflower And Leek Soup	34
Chicken And Vegetable Stew With Mushrooms	34

CHAPTER 6
SALADS — 35

Spinach And Berries Salad	36
Zucchini And Corn Salad	36
Tuna And Egg Salad With Olives	36
Crunchy Cabbage & Pumpkin Seed Slaw	36
Citrus Black Bean Quinoa Salad	37
Beetroot And Blackberry Salad With Tofu And Seeds	37
Pear And Walnut Salad	37
Chicken, Brussels Sprouts & Mushroom Salad	37
Kale, Avocado And Sweet Potato Bowl	38
Mediterranean Chickpea And Cucumber Salad	38
Asian Sesame Noodle Salad	39
Grilled Peach And Ricotta Salad	39
Turkey Cobb Salad	39
Watercress Salad	39
Thai Papaya Salad	40
The Ultimate Arugula & Feta Salad	40
Minted Lentil And Cucumber Salad	40
Edamame And Seaweed Salad	40

YOUR FREE GIFT
ANTI-INFLAMMATORY DIET BONUS BOOKS — **41**

CHAPTER 7
BREAKFASTS — 42

Oatmeal With Flaxseeds And Blueberries	43
Crispy Sweet Potato And Black Bean Skillet	43
Quick Chia Seeds Pudding With Berries	43
Coconut Yogurt Parfait With Berries And Walnuts	43
Vegan Pancakes With Orange Zest And Chocolate Chips	44
Miso Glazed Eggplant And Rice Breakfast Bowl	44
Chickpea Flour Crepes With Spiced Veggies	44
Avocado Toast With Turmeric & Hemp Seeds	44
Apple Cinnamon Quinoa Porridge	44
Herb-Infused Poached Eggs On Mushroom Toast	45
Pineapple Smoothie With Turmeric	45
Avocado And Pomegranate Salad Wrap	45
Sweet Potato Hash With Spinach	45
Savory Chickpea Pancakes With Spinach	45
Quinoa Breakfast Bowl With Almonds And Pomegranate	46
Tomato And Basil Baked Eggs With Artichokes	46
Curried Tofu Scramble	46

CHAPTER 8
FISH AND SEAFOOD — 47

Baked Grouper With Roasted Vegetables	48
Thai Coconut Curry Fish	48
Seared Scallops With Garlic Spinach	48
Spicy Grilled Mackerel	48
Pesto Baked Salmon	49
Garlic Parmesan Baked Tilapia	49
Blackened Fish Tacos	49
Sesame Ginger Grilled Trout	49
Sardines In Tomato Sauce	50
Spicy Crab Meat Stuffed Peppers	50
Spicy Crispy Calamari With Lime Dip	50
Baked Herb Crusted Halibut	50
Chili Garlic Mussels In Tomato Broth	50
Sea Bass With Greek Salad	51
Lemongrass Fish Skewers	51
Tuna Salad Lettuce Wraps	51
Grilled Salmon With Avocado Salsa	52
Shrimp Stir-Fry With Vegetables	52
Lemon Garlic Baked Thyme Cod	52
Creole Fish Stew	52

CHAPTER 9
MEAT AND POULTRY — 53

Golden Grilled Chicken	54
Herb-Citrus Turkey Skewers	54
Cilantro-Lime Grilled Pork Chops	54
Herb Crusted Chicken Cutlets	54
Honey Mustard Chicken Drumsticks	55
Sweet And Sour Turkey Meatballs	55
Ground Beef Stir-Fry	55
Harissa Roasted Lamb Meatballs	55
Peppercorn Crusted Steak With Garlic Butter	55
Spiced Moroccan Ground Lamb	55
Thai Coconut Curry Chicken	56
Cumin-Spiced Beef Tacos	56
Honey Garlic Chicken Thighs	56
Lemon-Herb Lamb Chops	57
Paprika-Rubbed Steak	57
Balsamic Glazed Chicken Breasts	57
Garlic Rosemary Pork Tenderloin	57

CHAPTER 10
EGGS AND GRAINS — 58

Quinoa Breakfast Bowl With Poached Eggs And Avocado	59
Zucchini Quinoa Frittata	59
Stuffed Egg Wrap With Minced Pork And Vegetables	59
Scrambled Egg And Farro Pilaf	59
Ramen With Soft-Boiled Egg And Tofu	60
Sweet Corn Egg Risotto	60
Egg And Millet Bowl With Spinach	60
Creamy Bacon & Egg Spaghetti	60
Spicy Egg And Couscous Bowl	61
Sorghum Egg Stir-Fry	61
Egg And Teff Porridge With Spices And Nuts	61

Creamy Polenta With Soft-Boiled Eggs	61
Parsley Bulgur Tabbouleh	61
Egg And Buckwheat Porridge	62
Shakshuka With Lentils And Herbs	62
Fluffy Omelette Rice	62
Egg And Barley Pilaf With Dried Fruits	63
Moroccan Scrambled Eggs With Crusty Bread	63
Mushroom And Scrambled Barley Risotto	63
Spinach and Feta Egg Muffins	63

CHAPTER 11
VEGETABLES — 64

Stuffed Acorn Squash With Lentils And Pomegranate	65
Cauliflower And Chickpea Curry	65
Roasted Turnips And Carrots With Mustard	65
Sauteed Belgium Endives With Oranges	65
Stuffed Bell Peppers With Quinoa And Black Beans	66
Roasted Root Vegetable Medley With Herbs	66
Cabbage Stir-Fry With Ginger And Carrots	66
Butternut Squash And Brussels Sprouts With Maple-Dijon Glaze	66
Korean-Style Tofu And Vegetables With Ginger Garlic Sauce	67
Garlic Butter Asparagus With Lemon Zest	67
Stewed Vegetable With Tofu And Mushrooms	67
Crispy Baked Artichoke Hearts	67
Turmeric Roasted Cauliflower	68
Hearty Vegetable Stew	68
Ginger-Garlic Sautéed Spinach	68
Grilled Zucchini And Eggplant With Lemon Tahini Sauce	68
Caramelized Anti-Inflammatory Vegetables	69
Spicy Sweet Potato Fries	69
Zucchini Noodles With Pesto	69
Roasted Parsnips With Lime And Cilantro	69

CHAPTER 12
SAUCES, CONDIMENTS AND DRESSINGS — 70

Beetroot Cashew Sauce	71
Creamy Basil Avocado Sauce	71
Walnut Parsley Pesto	71
Raspberry Vinaigrette	71
Zesty Chimichurri Sauce	72
Sesame Ginger Sauce	72
Pomegrante Mint Sauce	72
Spicy Coconut Sauce	72
Sweet Chilli Dipping Sauce	73
Almond Butter And Ginger Dip	73
Creamy Cashew Garlic Sauce	73
Homemade Tomato Ketchup	74
Lemon-Turmeric Vinaigrette	74
Tamarind Sauce	74
Ginger-Soy Dressing	74
Avocado-Cilantro Sauce	75
Green Goddess Dressing	75
Turmeric-Tahini Dressing	75
Spicy Mango Chutney	75
Garlic Dill Sauce	75

CHAPTER 13
SNACKS & QUICK BITES — 76

Walnuts And Dark Chocolate Bite	77
Roasted Pumpkin With Thyme	77
Avocado-Stuffed Sweet Potato Boats	77
Zucchini Pizza Bites	77
Tropical Berry Bliss Yogurt Bowl	78
Matcha Coconut Bliss Balls	78
Crispy Sushi Rolls	78
Turmeric Hummus With Veggie Sticks	79
Avocado And Berry Smoothie	79
Golden Milk Latte	79
Blueberry Almond Butter Cake	79
Sweet Pepper Guacamole Cups	79
Spiced Sweet Potato And Lentil Cakes	80
Anti-Inflammatory Green Smoothie	80
Mango Chia Pudding	80
Tahini Banana Rice Cakes	80

CHAPTER 14
DESSERTS — 81

- Spiced Baked Pears With Walnuts — 82
- Strawberry Coconut Ice Cream — 82
- Cinnamon Sweet Potato Brownies — 82
- Turmeric Coconut Energy Balls — 82
- No-Bake Lemon Cheesecake — 83
- Mango Banana Smoothie Bowl — 83
- Apple Cinnamon Cookies — 83
- Blueberry Cashew Cheesecake Bites — 84
- Raspberry Macaroons — 84
- Chocolate Covered Strawberries With Matcha — 84
- Chocolate Banana Muffins — 84
- Avocado Chocolate Mousse — 85
- Dark Chocolate Almond Bark — 85
- Coconut Popsicles — 85
- Pumpkin Spice Energy Bites — 85
- Almond Fudge Bars — 85

CHAPTER 15
FERMENTED FOODS — 86

- Mixed Vegetable Pickles — 87
- Labneh With Pita Bread — 87
- Tropical Pineapple Kombucha — 87
- Quick Stuffed Artichokes With Rice — 88
- Ginger-Glazed Tempeh — 88
- Fermented Berry And Lavender Infused Water — 88
- Miso Soup With Tempeh And Zucchini — 89
- Tangy Sauerkraut Slaw — 89
- Beetroot Yogurt Smoothie — 89
- Kefir Kiwi Bowl — 89
- Kimchi Fried Rice With Seaweed And White Sesame — 90
- Watermelon Fermented Salsa — 90
- Creamy Sourdough Toast With Cherries — 90
- Fermented Carrot And Ginger Pickle — 91
- Anti-Inflammatory Pickled Beets With Apple Cider Vinegar — 91
- Kimchi-Infused Veggie Stir-Fry — 91
- Anti-Inflammatory Ginger Turmeric Kombucha Smoothie — 91

MEAL PLAN 1-7 DAYS — 92

MEAL PLAN 8-15 DAYS — 93

MEAL PLAN 16-23 DAYS — 94

MEAL PLAN 24-30 DAYS — 95

CONVERSIONS AND EQUIVALENTS — 96

CONCLUSION — 97

THANK YOU — 98

REFERENCES — 99

INDEX — 100

INTRODUCTION

Welcome to your complete guide to a more self-empowered and healthier life! If you're new to this, you're about to embark on a crucial journey toward vitality and health.

Chronic inflammation is one of the biggest, yet often overlooked, threats to our health today. Recent studies indicate that around 60% of adults worldwide suffer from at least one chronic inflammatory condition—a statistic that reflects the rising prevalence of these health issues due to modern-day pressures, processed diets, and environmental pollutants (Global Burden of Disease Study, 2020).

This book, *The Practical Science-Backed Anti-Inflammatory Diet Cookbook for Beginners: Step by Step Plan, 200+ Super Easy Recipes & A 30-Day Meal Plan To Reset Your Cells, Immunity, and Gut Health and Ease Chronic Pain*, is designed to make the journey toward healing and wellness both meaningful and enjoyable, offering clear, actionable steps along the way.

The science behind this diet has been simplified, making it easy to understand the "why" and "how" of the healing process. Alongside foundational principles of the diet, this book features a volume of more than 200 quick and easy yet delicious, 30-minute recipes that bring the principles of the diet to life.

So, why embrace this approach? Research from *The American Journal of Clinical Nutrition* shows that diets rich in anti-inflammatory foods can significantly lower markers of inflammation and decrease the risk of conditions like heart disease, cancer, and diabetes.

In this book, you'll learn a step by step approach to listen to your own body and review your current diet. Chapter 4, *"Embracing an Anti-Inflammatory Diet: A Practical Guide,"* guides you to recognize trigger foods, find effective substitutes, and craft a diet that suits your unique needs.

Through the recipes and insights shared, you'll be able to take meaningful steps toward reducing inflammation, enhancing your microbiome, supporting cell rejuvenation, and boosting gut and brain health for a healthier, more balanced diet.

To make your journey even easier, check out these additional resources that are offered to you as bonus eBooks:

- 50 Powerful Anti-Inflammatory Ingredients Guidebook
- 45 Strategic Anti-Inflammatory Dietary & Stress Management Practices
- A Handbook of 100 Classic Anti-Inflammatory Recipes with Full Colored Pictures

I hope this book inspires and guides you on the journey to a healthier, happier and vibrant you. There's no time like the present to start this transformative journey. Let's get started on this exciting journey together!

A STEP BY STEP GUIDE: AN OVERVIEW ON HOW TO USE THIS ANTI-INFLAMMATORY DIET COOKBOOK

1. Adopt a Loving & Curious Mindset
Healing starts from within. Trust the process, give your best, and focus on small, consistent steps for lasting changes.

2. Understand the Basics (Chap. 1-3)
Learn why and how an anti-inflammatory diet works. This understanding will help you make choices that nourish and heal your body.

3. Assess Your Current Diet
Honestly evaluate your eating habits. Identify foods like processed snacks or fried items that might not serve your health well.

4. Implement an Elimination Diet (Chap. 4)

- **Practice Mindfulness:** Notice how foods make you feel during and after eating.
- **Remove Trigger Foods:** Use this chapter to identify and eliminate foods causing inflammation. Aim for at least 28 days but listen to your body.
- **Reintroduce Trigger Foods Gradually:** Slowly bring back these foods in moderation while noting how your body responds.

5. Explore the Recipes
Discover simple, delicious recipes that reduce inflammation. Look for alternatives to Trigger Foods and use the index for quick navigation.

6. Follow the 30-Day Meal Plan
Use the step-by-step meal plan for guidance. Each recipe is labeled for dietary preferences like gluten-free or vegan.

7. Use the Shopping Lists
Weekly lists make grocery trips easy and ensure you stick to anti-inflammatory ingredients.

8. Prep Ahead
Save time by preparing meals in advance. This keeps you on track even on busy days and reduces the temptation to eat less healthy foods.

9. Keep a Journal and Track Your Progress
Record changes in digestion, energy, and mood. Use your journal to guide reintroducing foods like eggs or gluten-free grains.

10. Incorporate Lifestyle Changes
Combine anti-inflammatory eating with regular movement, stress management, and good sleep for balanced healing.

11. Maintain Consistency
This is not a quick fix but a long-term lifestyle. Stick to the tools in this book to feel healthier and stronger over time.

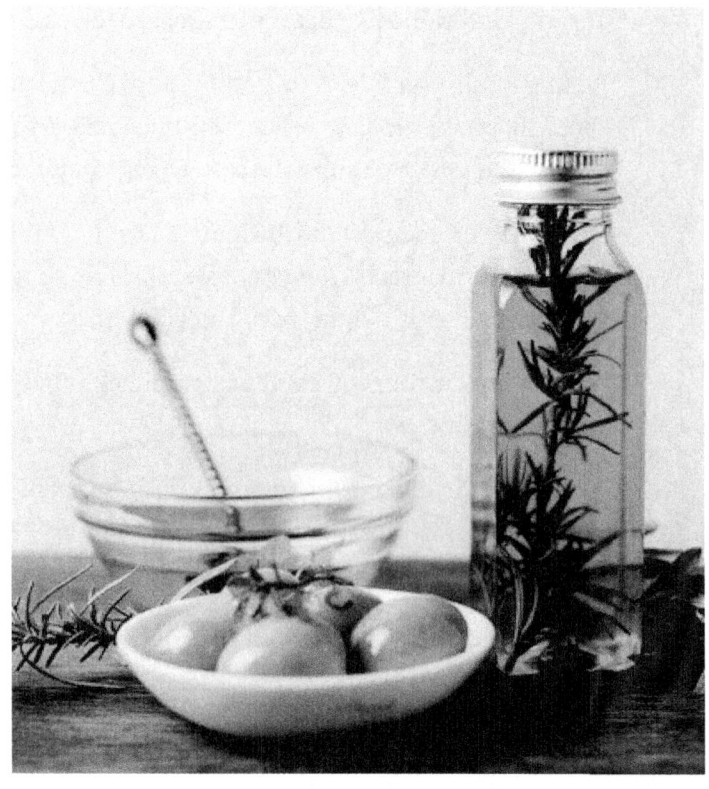

PURPOSE OF THE ANTI-INFLAMMATORY DIET COOKBOOK

This guide is designed to help you feel good from the inside out by addressing both the *why* and the *how* of an anti-inflammatory diet. Understanding the science behind inflammation and healing empowers you to make informed choices, while thoughtfully crafted recipes bring these principles to life.

The book starts by explaining how food and your body work together, highlighting why specific ingredients and methods support healing. This deeper understanding helps connect the diet to your wellness goals in a bigger, more meaningful way.

With balanced, easy-to-make recipes, practical tips, and a hassle-free 30-day meal plan, this book simplifies your journey. By making small, mindful changes, you can reduce inflammation, boost energy, and improve your overall well-being.

Inflammation is a part of life that can lead to fatigue, joint pain, and long-term health issues—but choosing the right foods can make a big difference.

Let this book be your trusted companion on your journey to better eating, and remember that choosing the right food is the foundation of good health.

Savour every delicious yet life-giving meal that enhance the sacredness of your well-being!

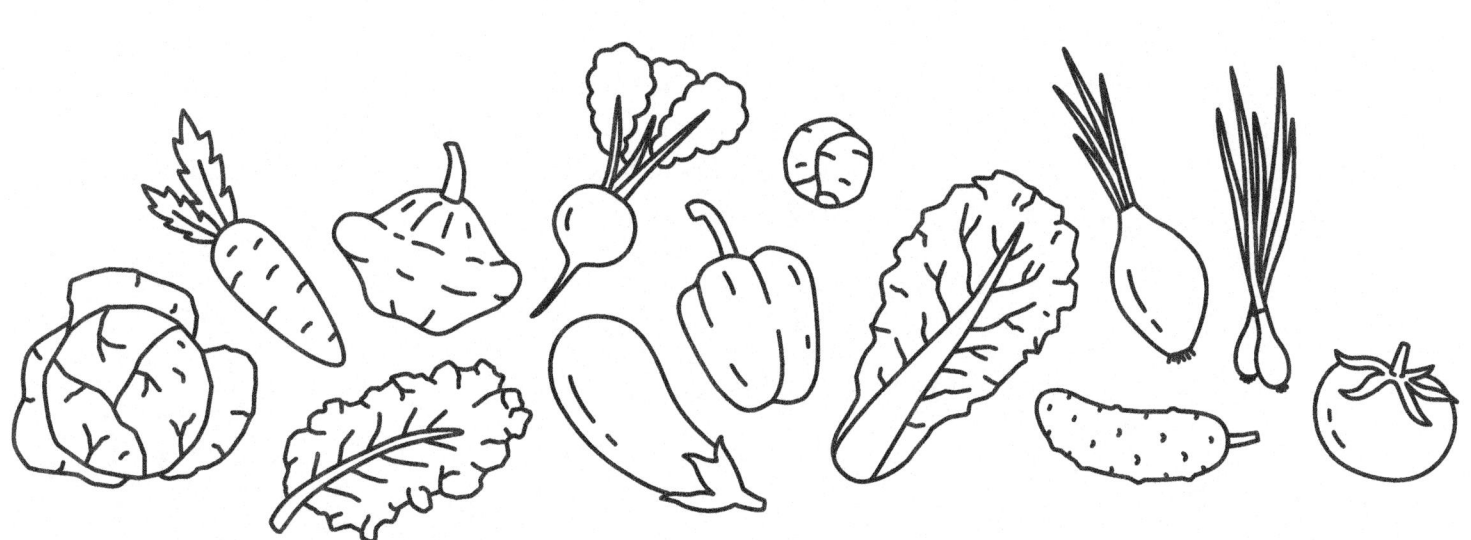

A PERSONAL JOURNEY
FROM PAIN TO EMPOWERMENT THROUGH FOOD

Hi, I'm Elena Florenz. For over 30 years, I worked in the food industry, creating delicious meals for people to enjoy. But my life took an unexpected turn when I faced some serious health problems. Like many people, I spent long hours working, often forgetting to take care of myself—until my health forced me to stop and pay attention.

It began with a simple fall. I thought I'd recover quickly, but I didn't. My joints became stiff and painful, making everyday tasks, like folding laundry, difficult. That's when I knew I had to make some changes. I took a step back from my career and started focusing on my health.

Not long after, I was diagnosed with gastritis, a painful condition where the stomach lining becomes inflamed. This diagnosis made me realize how important it is to pay attention to what I eat. I understood that true healing starts from within.

Food had always been my passion, but now it became my medicine. I learned which foods made me feel better, like almonds, millet, and figs, and which ones made my symptoms worse, like coffee and fried food. Even how I cooked my food mattered—steamed veggies became a gentle, comforting choice for my sensitive stomach.

Through this journey, I discovered that everyone's body is different. What helps one person might not work for another, and that's okay. But we can all learn to listen to our bodies and make choices that support our health.

This experience changed the way I think about food, and it inspired me to share recipes that not only taste great but also help with inflammation and support overall wellness. If you're struggling with inflammation, there's hope. You don't have to give up tasty food to feel better. You can enjoy meals that are both healing to the body and pleasing to the palate.

My goal is that these recipes make your journey to better health a little easier and a lot more enjoyable. Food isn't just fuel—it's a way to care for yourself.

Join me in discovering the balance, healing, and joy that can be found in your own kitchen to heal your body.

CHAPTER 1

ANTI-INFLAMMATORY DIET

"Healing begins on your plate, with each bite transforming into a mini super powerhouse to fight inflammation."

UNDERSTANDING THE ANTI-INFLAMMATORY DIET

The anti-inflammatory diet focuses on reducing inflammation in the body by choosing foods that have natural anti-inflammatory effects and avoiding those that promote inflammation.

The goal is to eat whole, nutrient-dense foods rich in antioxidants, vitamins, minerals, and healthy fats. But remember, it's not just a quick fix! Giving your body time to heal and rejuvenate is key. When you stick with it over the long haul, you'll find yourself feeling healthier and more vibrant in your daily life.

GOING BACK TO ANCIENT ROOTS

Anti-inflammatory diets have deep roots in ancient civilizations, where people naturally consumed whole, nutrient-dense foods known for their health benefits, long before processed foods became widespread.

Historical Roots:

- **Mediterranean Diet:**
  Countries like Greece and Italy emphasized fresh vegetables, fruits, fish, and healthy fats, with olive oil playing a key role in reducing inflammation due to its monounsaturated fats and antioxidants.

- **Traditional Asian Diets:**
  In regions like India and China, foods such as ginger, turmeric, garlic, and green tea were used not only for flavor but for their anti-inflammatory properties, thanks to their bioactive compounds.

- **Indigenous Diets:**
  Indigenous diets across the Americas and Africa were based on whole, unprocessed foods like legumes, nuts, and fresh produce, which supported balanced health and reduced inflammation.

The Link Between Diet and Inflammation

Chronic inflammation contributes to diseases such as heart disease, diabetes, and some cancers. Research shows that certain foods can either promote or reduce inflammation.

1. **Pro-Inflammatory Foods:**

Refined sugars, processed meats, and trans fats are major contributors to chronic inflammation. These foods can disrupt your body's natural balance, leading to increased inflammation and a higher risk of conditions like heart disease, diabetes, and joint pain. Minimizing their presence in your diet is the first step to reducing inflammation.

2. **Anti-Inflammatory Foods:**

- Incorporate a variety of antioxidant-rich, nutrient-dense foods, such as leafy greens, berries, whole grains, legumes, nuts, seeds, and fatty fish. These foods help lower inflammation and promote overall health.

- Prioritize plant-based options like fruits, vegetables, and whole grains, as they are naturally packed with compounds that combat inflammation effectively.

EATING PATTERNS FOR ANTI-INFLAMMATORY DIET

Balancing macronutrients is key to reducing inflammation and supporting overall health.

- **Vitamins and Minerals**: Promote energy, mental clarity, mood stability, and recovery from stress or injuries.
- **Carbohydrates**: Provide steady energy, control hunger, and boost positivity when consumed in limited amounts.
- **Proteins**: Aid in brain health, mental clarity, injury recovery, and anti-aging, while fostering overall well-being.
- **Fats and Oils**: Support brain structure, mood regulation, chronic disease prevention, and good health through healthy fat sources.

Together, these components create a solid foundation for a sustainable anti-inflammatory lifestyle.

Food Group	Servings per Day	Serving Size	Examples
Vegetables 30%	4–5 servings	1 cup raw or ½ cup cooked	Spinach, broccoli, bell peppers, carrots
Fruits 15%	2–4 servings	1 medium fruit or ½ cup chopped	Berries, apples, oranges, cherries
Whole Grains 20%	3–4 servings	½ cup cooked or 1 slice whole-grain bread	Brown rice, quinoa, oats
Healthy Fats 10%	2–3 servings	1 tbsp olive oil, ¼ cup nuts, 2 tbsp seeds	Olive oil, almonds, chia seeds, avocado
Lean Proteins 15%	2–3 servings	3–4 oz fish/poultry or ½ cup plant protein	Salmon, chicken, tofu, lentils
Dairy/Alternatives 5%	1–2 servings	1 cup low-fat yogurt or dairy-free alt.	Greek yogurt, almond milk
Hydration 5%	8–10 glasses	8 oz per glass	Water, herbal teas

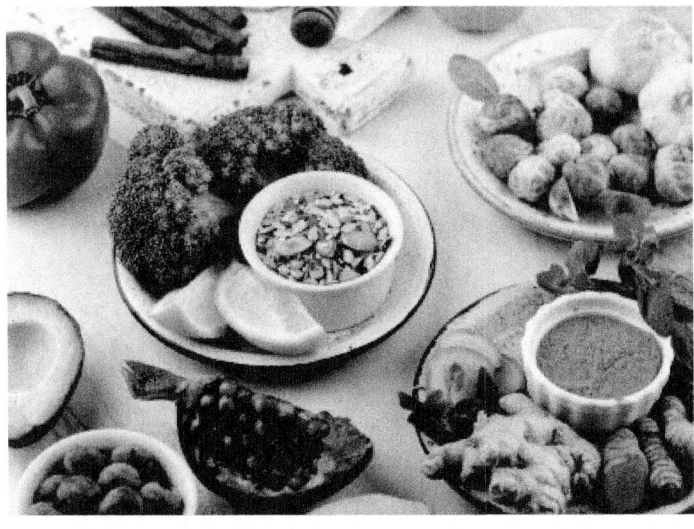

HOW STAYING HYDRATED HELPS WITH PAIN AND INFLAMMATION

Our bodies are 97% water, and we need it to function properly. Water helps flush out toxins and keep tissues like joints lubricated. When we're dehydrated, joints lose lubrication, causing pain and inflammation. Drinking water also boosts synovial fluid, which helps joints move smoothly.

Staying hydrated can be difficult sometimes, but these simple tips can help:

- **Start Your Morning Hydrated**
  Begin with a glass of water as soon as you wake up to refresh your body. Keep a glass or bottle by your bedside as a gentle reminder each morning.

- **Track Your Water Progress**
  Jot down your daily intake to notice any positive shifts in your energy, skin, or joint health. Gradually increasing your intake could help with any inflammation or discomfort.

- **Set Realistic Hydration Goals**
  Aim for one glass per hour or with each meal to make hydration a habit. Try swapping sugary drinks for water, and infuse your water with lemon, cucumber, or mint for a refreshing twist, making hydration feel less like a chore and more like a treat.

- **Use Gentle Reminders**
  Set reminders on your phone or fitness tracker, or place sticky notes in spots you frequent to prompt a quick drink.

- **Always Keep A Water Bottle Handy**
  Bring a water bottle with you, whether at home, work, or out and about. It makes staying hydrated easier throughout the day.

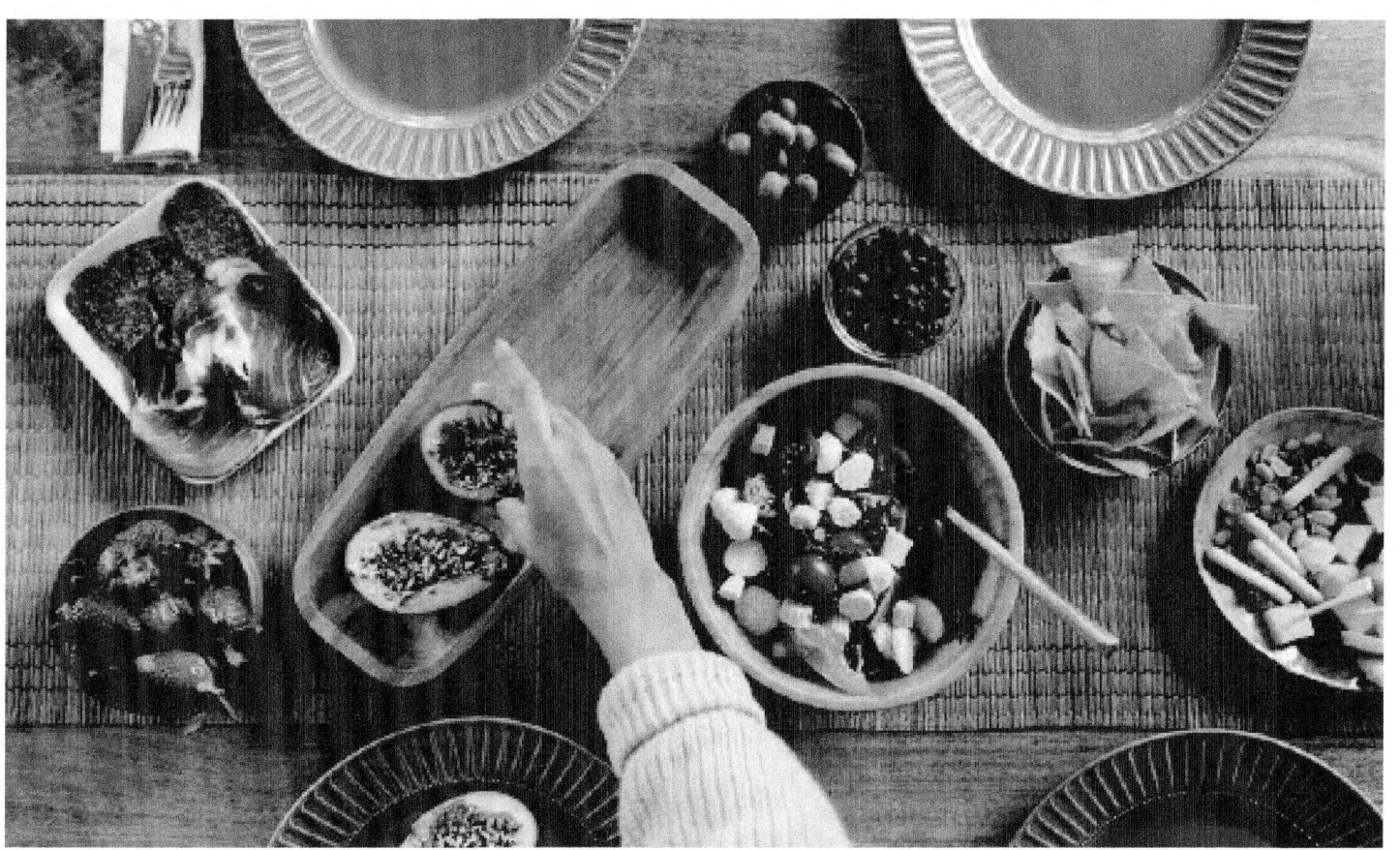

CHAPTER 2

GETTING TO KNOW INFLAMMATION

"Rebuild from within—cell by cell, and observe your health bloom."

HOW INFLAMMATION WORKS THROUGH OUR IMMUNE SYSTEM

Ever wondered why your body feels pain, swelling, or stiffness? That's inflammation at work!

It's your body's natural defense, stepping in to protect you from harm like infections or injuries. When something harmful is detected, your immune system triggers inflammation to heal and protect the affected area.

Here's how it works: Your immune cells release chemicals like bradykinin and histamine, causing blood vessels to widen. This allows more blood to flow to the area, making it red and warm.

The extra blood brings immune cells to help with healing. But these chemicals also stimulate nerves, which send pain signals to your brain, making inflammation feel painful.

It's your body's way of telling you to rest and give the area time to heal.

TYPES OF INFLAMMATION

Inflammation is like your body's alarm system—It's designed to protect you. Acute inflammation is the good kind: it kicks in quickly to heal injuries or fight infections. It's temporary, and once the job's done, it leaves. But chronic inflammation is the troublemaker. When it lingers too long, it starts to damage your tissues, increasing the risk of diseases like arthritis, heart disease, and even gut issues.

Aspect	Acute Inflammation	Chronic Inflammation
What is it?	A short-term, immediate response to injury or infection; lasts from hours to days	A long-term, persistent response that can last for months or even years
Cause	Triggered by infections, injuries, or irritants	Triggered by prolonged irritants, unresolved acute inflammation, autoimmune responses, or hormonal changes (e.g., menopause)
Signs	Redness, warmth, swelling, pain, and loss of function in the affected area	Subtle signs like joint pain, fatigue, digestive issues, skin changes, and body aches

Aspect	Acute Inflammation	Chronic Inflammation
Inflammation: Good or Bad?	Good - Helps the body heal by increasing blood flow, immune cells, and nutrients to the affected area	Bad - Persistent inflammation can harm tissues and organs, leading to disease
Effects on the Body	Initiates healing and protects the body; encourages rest to prevent further injury	Causes tissue damage over time, increasing the risk for chronic diseases and cellular stress
Associated Diseases	Usually temporary; resolves on its own or with treatment (e.g., infections, minor injuries)	Linked to conditions like arthritis, heart disease, diabetes, cancer, Alzheimer's, gut health issues (e.g., IBS), and menopausal symptoms
Cellular-Level Impact	Minimal long-term impact on cells, as inflammation subsides once healing occurs	Ongoing cellular stress, leading to oxidative stress, DNA damage, and weakened immunity

HOW INFLAMMATION AFFECTS THE HUMAN BODY

Before diving into the role of diet in managing inflammation, it's essential to understand how inflammation impacts various parts of the body. The following illustration highlights the widespread effects of chronic inflammation on organs and systems—from the brain to the heart, muscles, and beyond. Recognizing these impacts can empower you to make informed choices to support your body's healing.

See how inflammation affects different areas and the health issues it can lead to over time.

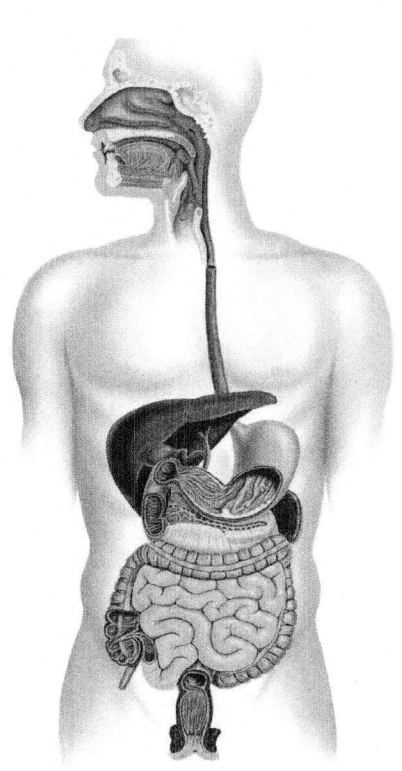

BRAIN
Pro-inflammatory cytokines cause autoimmune reactions in the brain. Leads to depression, autism, poor memory, Alzheimer's disease, and Multiple Sclerosis (MS).

CARDIOVASCULAR
Inflammation in the heart, arterial, and venous walls contributes to heart disease, stroke, high blood sugar (diabetes), and anemia.

MUSCLE
Inflammatory cytokines cause muscle pain and weakness. Can manifest as carpal tunnel syndrome or polymyalgia rheumatica.

BONES
Inflammation interferes with natural bone repair, increasing fracture risk and leading to osteoporosis.

SKIN
Chronic inflammation affects the liver and kidneys, resulting in rashes, dermatitis, eczema, acne, psoriasis, wrinkles, and fine lines.

THYROID
Autoimmunity caused by inflammation reduces thyroid receptor count and disrupts thyroid hormone function.

LUNGS
Inflammation triggers autoimmune reactions in airway linings, causing allergies or asthma.

GI TRACT
Chronic inflammation damages intestinal lining and causes GERD, Crohn's disease, and Celiac disease.

KIDNEYS
Inflammatory cytokines restrict blood flow to the kidneys, leading to edema, hypertension, nephritis, and kidney failure.

LIVER
Inflammation causes liver enlargement or fatty liver disease, increasing toxic load build-up in the body.

KEY INFLAMMATORY HEALTH CONDITIONS & THEIR SUPPORTING FOODS

We know that chronic inflammation can have a profound effect on your life, creating a restricted lifestyle and leading to a variety of health challenges. It can both cause and be caused by certain conditions. Here are some common issues associated with inflammation:

Category	Impact on Inflammation	Health Effects	Supporting Foods
Neurological	Inflammatory foods increase brain inflammation.	Memory loss, brain fog, depression, dementia, Alzheimer's, Parkinson's, anxiety, cognitive decline	Berries, leafy greens, fatty fish, turmeric, walnuts, olive oil
Cardiovascular	Processed foods and trans fats increase heart inflammation.	High blood pressure, heart disease, stroke, atherosclerosis, arrhythmias, heart attack, coronary artery disease	Olive oil, nuts, seeds, green tea, berries, leafy greens
Digestive	Poor diet damages gut lining, causing digestive inflammation.	Bloating, IBS, constipation, acid reflux, Crohn's disease, ulcerative colitis, leaky gut syndrome	Yogurt, ginger, garlic, fiber-rich foods, kefir, leafy greens
Gut Health	Chronic gut inflammation leads to systemic inflammation.	Leaky gut, dysbiosis, IBS, IBD, chronic digestive discomfort	Probiotics, prebiotics, fiber, bone broth, omega-3s, turmeric
Metabolic	Sugar and refined carbs cause insulin resistance and inflammation.	Obesity, insulin resistance, type 2 diabetes, metabolic syndrome, fatty liver disease	Whole grains, legumes, vegetables, berries, avocado, olive oil
Immune System	Inflammatory foods weaken immune response, promoting autoimmune diseases.	Rheumatoid arthritis, lupus, multiple sclerosis, psoriasis, other autoimmune disorders	Citrus fruits, bell peppers, almonds, turmeric, leafy greens, fatty fish
Others	Chronic inflammation affects organs, increasing disease risk.	Cancer, osteoporosis, asthma, chronic pain, COPD, liver diseases, kidney disease	Tomatoes, leafy greens, nuts, seeds, berries, ginger, green tea

CHAPTER 3

MICROBIOME, IMMUNE SYSTEM AND CELLULAR REGENERATION

"Rebuild from within—cell by cell, and observe your health bloom."

Your microbiome, immune system, and cellular regeneration are deeply interconnected, working together to maintain and restore your body's health.

The immune system acts as your body's protector, responding to threats like infections, injuries, or harmful invaders. Meanwhile, the microbiome—trillions of tiny microbes in your gut—serves as an ally, supporting the immune system and guiding cellular regeneration.

Cellular regeneration is the body's ability to repair, replace, or create new cells. This process is vital for healing wounds, recovering from illness, and maintaining healthy organs and tissues. Here's how it all connects:

1. **The Microbiome's Role**: A balanced microbiome nurtures your gut lining, reducing inflammation and sending signals to your immune system. These signals trigger proper immune responses, such as repairing damaged cells or targeting harmful invaders.

2. **Immune System Collaboration**: The immune system relies on the microbiome to identify threats while also regulating inflammation. When the immune system is overactive (as in chronic inflammation), the microbiome steps in to help calm it, giving the body a chance to regenerate healthy cells.

3. **Cellular Regeneration**: The microbiome produces metabolites like short-chain fatty acids, which fuel the gut lining and support cellular repair and regeneration. A healthy microbiome ensures a steady cycle of cell renewal, aiding recovery and long-term health.

When your gut health thrives, your immune system and cellular regeneration processes are optimized, allowing your body to rebuild from within—cell by cell. This balance is a cornerstone of an anti-inflammatory lifestyle.

WHY GUT HEALTH IS SO IMPORTANT FOR HEALING?

A healthy gut microbiome is super important because it can help control inflammation, reduce stress on your body, and support the healing process.

The microbes in your gut can produce short-chain fatty acids (SCFAs) like butyrate, which have anti-inflammatory properties. These SCFAs help maintain the lining of your gut, keeping harmful substances from leaking into your bloodstream and causing more inflammation.

When your gut is out of balance (a state called dysbiosis), it can lead to "leaky gut," where toxins and bacteria escape into your system, creating inflammation and slowing down your healing process.

HOW TO BUILD A GUT-FRIENDLY ANTI-INFLAMMATORY DIET?

A gut-friendly, anti-inflammatory diet focuses on nourishing the gut microbiome while reducing inflammation throughout the body.

Incorporating a balance of probiotics, prebiotics, fiber-rich foods, healthy fats, and antioxidant-rich ingredients can help restore gut health, improve digestion, and enhance overall well-being.

Here's a comprehensive table highlighting the key components of such a diet:

Category	Benefits	Examples	Role in Gut Health
Probiotic Foods	Introduces beneficial bacteria	Yogurt (lactose-free), kefir, kimchi, sauerkraut, kombucha	Restores gut flora, improves digestion, boosts immunity, reduces inflammation
Prebiotic Foods	Feeds beneficial bacteria, supports their growth	Garlic, bananas, onions, asparagus, Jerusalem artichokes	Stimulates growth of healthy bacteria, enhances gut health
Fiber-Rich Foods	Nourishes gut bacteria, promotes a healthy microbiome	Peas, apples, berries, broccoli, oats, lentils	Provides essential fuel for gut bacteria, supports digestion and gut diversity
Healthy Fats	Reduces inflammation, supports gut health	Salmon, walnuts, flaxseeds, chia seeds	Contains omega-3s that help balance gut bacteria and reduce inflammation
Polyphenol-Rich Foods	Offers antioxidant and anti-inflammatory effects	Dark chocolate, green tea, berries, spinach	Promotes beneficial bacteria growth, reduces oxidative stress
Fermented Foods	Enhances gut microbiome diversity	Sourdough, miso	Provides live beneficial bacteria to support gut function
Avoiding Pro-Inflammatory Foods	Protects gut and reduces inflammation	Processed foods, refined sugars, trans fats	Prevents microbial imbalance and chronic inflammation

THE IMPACT OF ULTRA-PROCESSED FOODS ON YOUR GUT HEALTH

Ever wonder why processed foods, like chips and packaged cookies, don't do your body any favors? These foods can harm your gut and overall health as they cause the following:

Gut Microbiota Disruption:

- **Reduced SCFAs:** Ultra-processed foods lower levels of beneficial short-chain fatty acids (SCFAs), which weakens the gut lining and increases gut permeability.

- **Inflammation:** A compromised gut lining allows harmful substances to enter the bloodstream, triggering inflammation.

Low Nutritional Quality:

- **High in Sugar and Unhealthy Fats:** These contribute to inflammation and disturb the gut's balance.
- **Low in Fiber and Nutrients:** Essential for feeding beneficial bacteria and supporting digestion, fiber and micronutrients are often lacking in processed foods.

Additives and Chemical Exposure:

- **Emulsifiers and Sweeteners:** These additives can disrupt gut bacteria and promote inflammation.
- **Harmful Chemicals:** Substances like bisphenol and phthalates from packaging or acrylamide from high-heat cooking can impair gut health.

Why It Matters: Chronic consumption of ultra-processed foods can lead to low-grade, persistent inflammation linked to conditions like heart disease and diabetes. Choosing whole, fresh foods supports gut health, reduces inflammation, and improves overall well-being. Opting for minimally processed foods helps maintain a healthier gut and reduces the risk of long-term health issues.

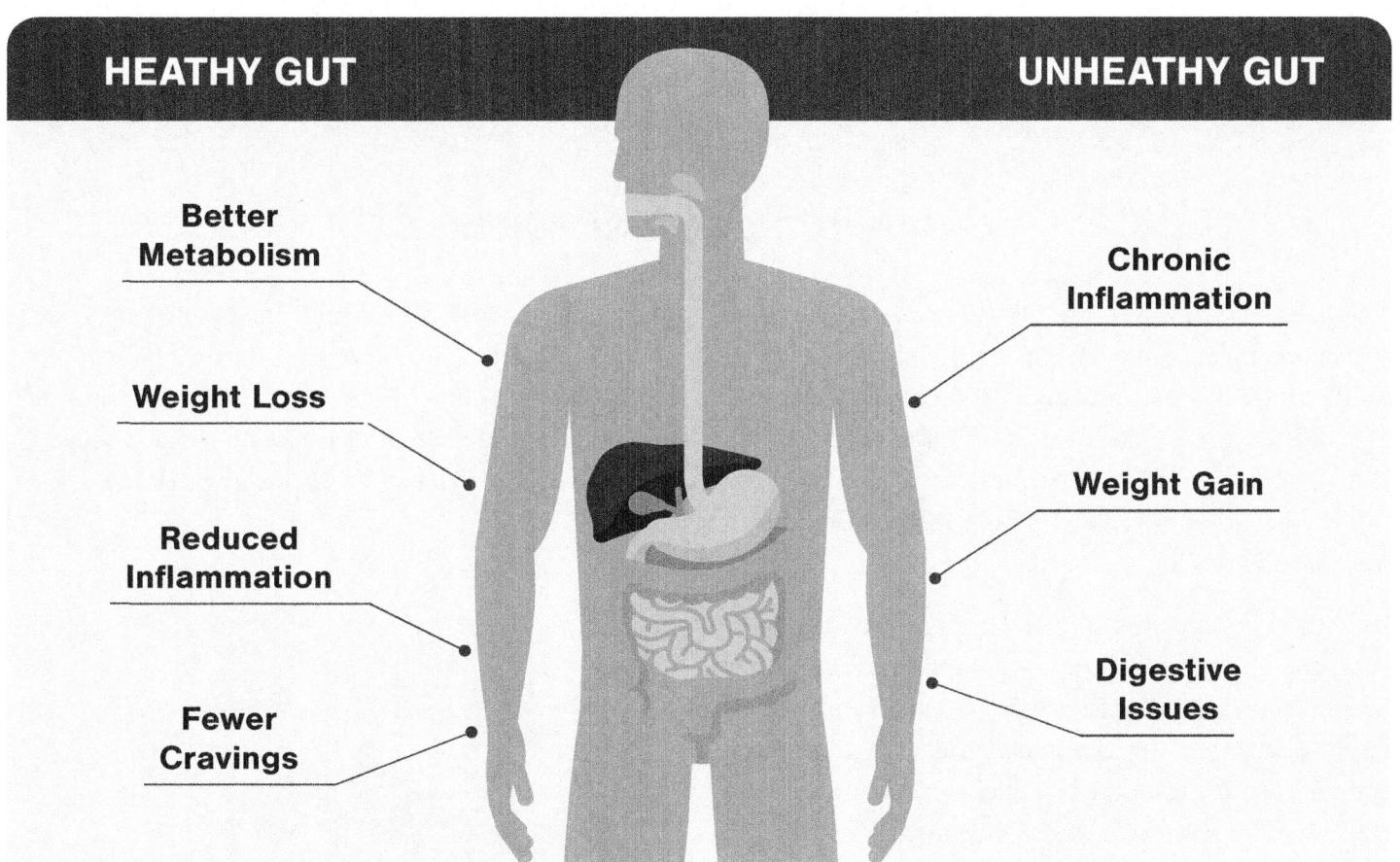

CHAPTER 4

EMBRACING AN ANTI-INFLAMMATORY DIET & LIFESTYLE: A PRACTICAL GUIDE

"Vitality lies in the foods that calm your body and energize your soul."

ADOPTING THE ELIMINATION DIET

This eating approach, known as the elimination diet, is a temporary plan designed to give the body a break from foods that may cause inflammation or damage to the gut. By cutting out foods that could lead to issues like "leaky gut" (increased gut permeability) and hormonal imbalances, this diet aims to help restore the body's natural balance.

Dr. Albert Rowe, an allergist, is often credited with advancing the systematic approach to elimination diets in his studies on food allergies and delayed hypersensitivities. He introduced structured methods to identify allergens by carefully removing and reintroducing foods, providing a scientific foundation for identifying dietary triggers and improving patient outcomes.

Many people today experience symptoms related to food sensitivities and gut issues, but these conditions are often underdiagnosed and misunderstood. Nutrition plays a powerful role in reducing inflammation in the body, allowing it to heal and function optimally without the strain of harmful foods and toxins.

The main goals of this elimination diet are to heal the gut lining, support a balanced gut microbiome (the community of beneficial organisms in our gut), reduce overall inflammation, and uncover any hidden food sensitivities. Throughout the process, it's essential to keep track of any symptoms in a food journal, which helps you understand how different foods affect your body.

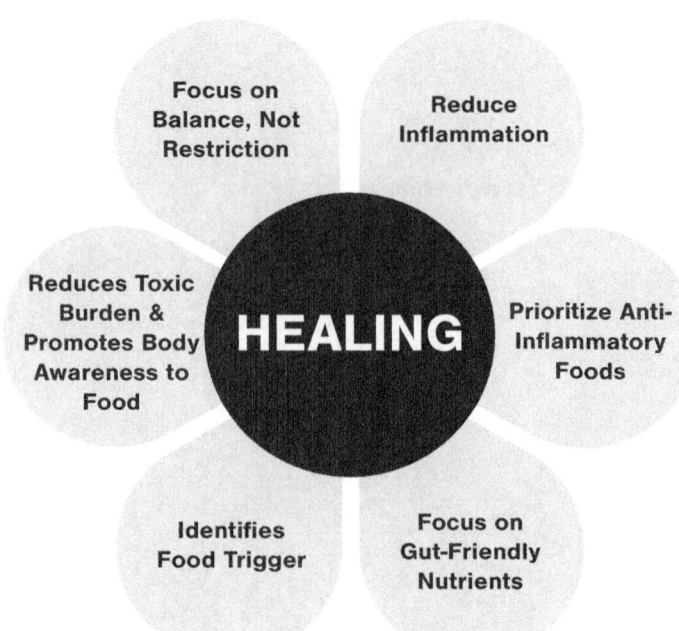

PLANNING THE ELIMINATION DIET

The elimination diet involves two primary stages: elimination and reintroduction. This structured approach helps you identify any food intolerances or triggers of inflammation in your diet.

1. Elimination Phase (28 Days):

In this stage, you'll avoid specific food groups that are common inflammation triggers.

Check out the *'Elimination Diet Food Guide'* below to learn which foods should be eliminated. You'll focus on whole foods, lean proteins, healthy fats, and low-glycemic fruits. It's essential to be strict with avoiding the foods that fall outside the allowed list during these 28 days.

To make your journey through the Elimination Phase effortless, be sure to check out the detailed 30-day meal plan created specifically for this stage.

It's packed with easy-to-follow recipes and meal ideas that align with the elimination guidelines, helping you stay on track while enjoying nourishing, delicious meals.

2. Reintroduction Phase:

After 28 days, the food listed in 'Foods to Avoid' in the table below are gradually reintroduced one group at a time, allowing you to observe any negative reactions.

Each group should be reintroduced over three days, with two days in between to monitor for any adverse symptoms like bloating, fatigue, or headaches.

Keep a detailed journal of:

- The food reintroduced
- The amount consumed
- Any symptoms observed
- How long symptoms lasted

Here's a suggested schedule for reintroducing each group:

1. **Days 1-3: Proteins** (beef, pork, eggs)
   Day 1: Reintroduce food one by one from this group, then monitor your body for symptoms on Days 2 and 3.

2. **Days 4-6: Dairy** (cheese, milk, yogurt)
   Reintroduce on Day 4, monitor for reactions on Days 5 and 6.

3. **Days 7-9: Gluten Grains** (bread, pasta)
   Reintroduce on Day 7, observe for any symptoms on Days 8 and 9.

4. **Days 10-12: Nightshade Vegetables** (tomatoes, peppers)
   Introduce these on Day 10 and monitor closely for inflammatory responses.

5. **Days 13-15: Beverages** (coffee, alcohol, green tea)
   Introduce these beverages on Day 13, watching for any reactions.

6. **Days 16-18: Fruits** (citrus, bananas, melons)
   Reintroduce on Day 16 and monitor for signs of intolerance.

7. **Days 19-21: Sugars** (honey, maple syrup)
   Introduce sugars on Day 19, observe for any adverse symptoms through Days 20 and 21.

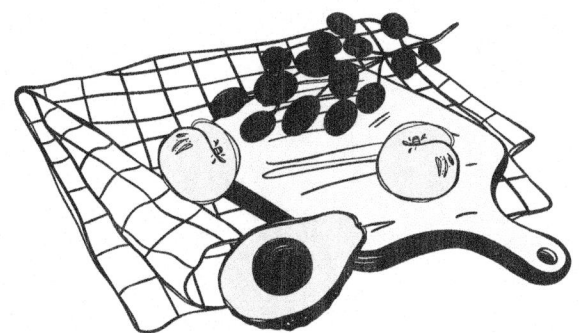

ELIMINATION DIET FOOD GUIDE

Food Groups	Allowed Foods	Foods to Avoid (First 28 Days)
Proteins Day 1-3	Poultry, lamb, bison, venison, cold-water fish (e.g., salmon, trout), legumes (beans, lentils)	Beef, pork, veal, processed meats (sausage, cold cuts), shellfish, eggs
Carbohydrates Day 7-9	Sweet potatoes, quinoa, buckwheat, brown rice	White potatoes, gluten-containing grains (wheat, barley, rye), baked goods, bread, pasta
Vegetables Day 10-12	All non-nightshade vegetables, especially cruciferous types like broccoli, cauliflower, kale	Nightshades (tomatoes, eggplant, white potatoes, peppers)
Fruits Day 16-18	Low-glycemic fruits like apples, berries, cherries, plums	High-glycemic or allergenic fruits (ripe bananas, pineapple, citrus), melon
Fats and Oils	Extra virgin olive oil, avocado oil, raw nuts (almonds, walnuts)	Refined oils, margarine, peanuts, peanut butter
Beverages Day 13-15	Filtered water, herbal teas (chamomile, peppermint)	Coffee, alcohol, sugary beverages, citrus juices, green tea
Dairy Products Day 4-6	None	Milk, cheese, yogurt, cream
Sweeteners Day 19-21	None	Table sugar, honey, artificial sweeteners (e.g., aspartame), maple syrup

FOOD SUBSTITUTIONS

Here is a list of substitutions for foods that you can opt while on the Elimination Diet.

If You Use This...	Replace It With This...	Why Choose This?
Milk (for cereal or shakes)	Coconut milk, macadamia milk, unsweetened oat milk, or flax milk. Ensure it's free from lactose, casein, and added sugars.	These options are dairy-free, easier to digest, and support gut health by avoiding common allergens.
Hot cereals (e.g., cream of wheat)	Quinoa porridge, millet pudding, or buckwheat groats with cinnamon and berries.	These alternatives are gluten-free, packed with fiber, and help maintain stable blood sugar levels.
Cold cereals	Gluten-free granola, toasted quinoa clusters, or amaranth flakes sweetened naturally with fruit.	Gluten-free cereals reduce inflammation and support better digestion for sensitive stomachs.
Bread, crackers, pasta	Sweet potato wraps, cassava crackers, zucchini noodles, or pasta made from chickpeas, lentils, or green peas.	These options are high in fiber and protein while being free from gluten, which can irritate the gut lining.

Quick breads	Almond flour banana bread, coconut flour pumpkin muffins, or spiced sweet potato pancakes.	These options use nutrient-dense flours and natural sweeteners to avoid gluten and refined sugar.
Breading	Crushed rice crackers, almond meal, ground flaxseeds, or coconut flour.	These alternatives create a crunchy coating while adding healthy fats and nutrients.
Eggs	Aquafaba (chickpea water), mashed banana, or a flaxseed egg (1 tbsp ground flax + 3 tbsp water).	Ideal for those avoiding eggs, these options provide binding and moisture without allergens.
Peanut butter	Sunflower seed butter, pumpkin seed butter, tahini, or almond butter.	These substitutes avoid common allergens like peanuts while providing healthy fats and minerals.
Ice cream	Coconut milk ice cream, frozen banana "nice cream," or avocado chocolate mousse.	These options are dairy-free and naturally sweetened, minimizing gut irritation and added sugar.
Soda and fizzy drinks	Sparkling water infused with berries, ginger kombucha, or herbal iced tea with lemon.	These choices avoid artificial sweeteners and high sugar content while offering hydration and digestive support.
Coffee/tea	Dandelion root coffee, golden milk (turmeric latte), or rooibos tea.	These caffeine-free options are gentle on the gut and packed with antioxidants.
Butter/margarine	Avocado oil, coconut oil, or ghee (if tolerated).	These fats are anti-inflammatory and free from hydrogenated oils found in margarine.
Sweeteners	Date paste, coconut sugar, pure maple syrup, or monk fruit sweetener.	These natural sweeteners have a lower glycemic impact and are less processed than refined sugar.
Condiments	Fresh pesto, tahini dressing, or homemade salsa with no added preservatives.	These options are nutrient-rich, free from additives, and promote better digestion.

GENERAL FOOD GUIDE

Here's a simple guide to help you choose foods that reduce inflammation and avoid those that can make it worse. Check out the table below for easy options!

Foods to Eat & Why They're Beneficial	Foods to Avoid & Why to Avoid
Salmon, Mackerel, Sardines: Rich in omega-3 fatty acids, reduce inflammation, especially for heart disease and arthritis.	**Refined Carbs (White Bread, Pastries):** Cause blood sugar spikes, leading to increased inflammation.
Spinach, Kale, Swiss Chard, Broccoli, Cauliflower: High in vitamins and antioxidants that reduce inflammation.	**Fried Foods (Fries, Fried Chicken):** High in trans fats and AGEs, promote inflammation.

Berries (Blueberries, Strawberries), Citrus (Oranges, Lemons): Antioxidants that lower chronic inflammation and oxidative stress.	**Processed Meats (Bacon, Sausage):** Contain preservatives and fats that increase inflammation.
Olive Oil (Extra Virgin), Avocados: Anti-inflammatory fats that support joint health and reduce oxidative stress.	**Sugary Beverages (Soda, Energy Drinks):** Excessive sugar consumption linked to chronic inflammation.
Turmeric, Ginger, Garlic: Anti-inflammatory compounds that support digestion, joint health, and immunity.	**Artificial Trans Fats (Margarine):** Linked to inflammation and heart disease.
Quinoa, Brown Rice, Oats: High in fiber, support gut health, and reduce inflammation.	**Excessive Alcohol:** Chronic alcohol consumption triggers inflammation and liver issues.
Almonds, Walnuts, Chia Seeds, Flaxseeds: High in healthy fats and omega-3s, reduce inflammation and promote heart health.	**Processed Snacks (Chips, Cookies):** High in refined flour, sugar, and unhealthy fats.
Lentils, Chickpeas, Black Beans: High in fiber and protein, reduce inflammation and support gut health.	**Refined Vegetable Oils (Soybean, Corn):** High omega-6 fatty acids, promote inflammation.
70% or Higher Dark Chocolate: Contains polyphenols that reduce inflammation and improve heart health.	**High-Sugar Desserts (Cakes, Ice Cream):** Excess sugar intake increases inflammatory markers.
Sweet Potatoes, Beets: Rich in fiber, vitamins, and antioxidants that reduce inflammation and improve blood flow.	**Processed Baked Goods (Cookies, Muffins):** Contain trans fats, sugar, and refined flour, contributing to inflammation.
Shiitake, Maitake Mushrooms: Antioxidants that protect against chronic disease and inflammation.	**Salty Processed Foods (Canned Goods):** High salt content can cause water retention and increase inflammation.

Benefits of the Elimination Diet

- **Personalized Insights:** This diet helps you discover personal food triggers.

- **Long-term Inflammation Control:** By identifying and avoiding foods that trigger inflammation, you can maintain improved health and keep these foods on your personal *watch list*. This awareness not only helps in controlling inflammation but also ensures better long-term health outcomes.

- **Positive Life Changes:** To achieve results require dedication, patience and consistency but the rewards of the valuable insights can be life-changing as you learn to manage inflammatory responses.

With this step-by-step approach, this elimination diet offers lasting benefits with minimal stress. where you are empowered to listen to your body and take the next steps to heal your body innately. Through this process, you'll regain control over your health by identifying food triggers and reducing inflammation in a sustainable way.

For readers with dietary preferences, we have marked each recipe as Vegan (VG), Vegetarian (V), Gluten Free (GF), Nut Free (NF), Dairy Free (DF) and Soy Free (SF) where applicable.

TIPS FOR STOCKING AND SOURCING INGREDIENTS:

- **Shop Local and Seasonal**: Local farmers' markets or co-ops often provide the freshest produce at reasonable prices. Seasonal fruits and vegetables are not only fresher but also often more affordable.

- **Buy in Bulk**: Grains, legumes, and nuts can be bought in bulk, saving you money and reducing packaging waste. Store them in airtight containers to maintain freshness.

- **Look for Organic and Non-GMO**: Prioritize organic, non-GMO produce, especially when buying high-pesticide items like berries and leafy greens (following the "Dirty Dozen" list).

- **Use Frozen Produce**: Frozen fruits and vegetables are often picked at peak ripeness and retain their nutrients. They're a great way to have anti-inflammatory staples available year-round.

- **Grow Your Own Herbs**: Fresh herbs like basil, rosemary, and cilantro are easy to grow at home, either in pots or a small garden, giving you a constant supply of anti-inflammatory flavors.

- **Prioritize Quality Oils**: Cold-pressed, extra-virgin olive oil and coconut oil are key sources of healthy fats. Always opt for high-quality oils, which can often be found in glass bottles to preserve their freshness. This setup helps you build a pantry that supports long-term anti-inflammatory eating.

DOWNLOAD YOUR BONUS
ANTI-INFLAMMATORY RECIPE BOOK WITH VIBRANT, FULL COLOR PICTURES

A HANDBOOK OF 100 CLASSIC ANTI-INFLAMMATORY RECIPES WITH FULL COLORED PICTURES

Let this delightful recipe booklet be your go-to reference guide. Each recipe features a special *Health Perks* section and *a full-colored photo* to help you identify the key elements of each food group so you can prepare more meals with confidence.

Get access to this vibrant and fun recipe booklet, and other bonus ebooks by copying the below link and pasting it in your browser or scanning the QR code with your mobile phone's camera.

https://heartbookspress.com/Anti-InflammatoryDietCookbook-FreeBonuses

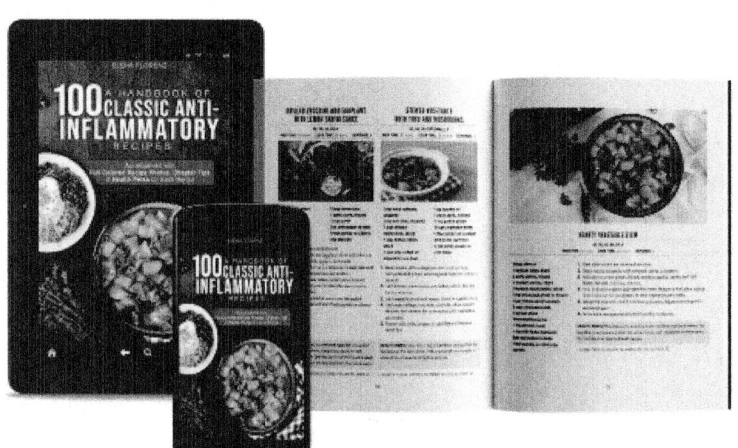

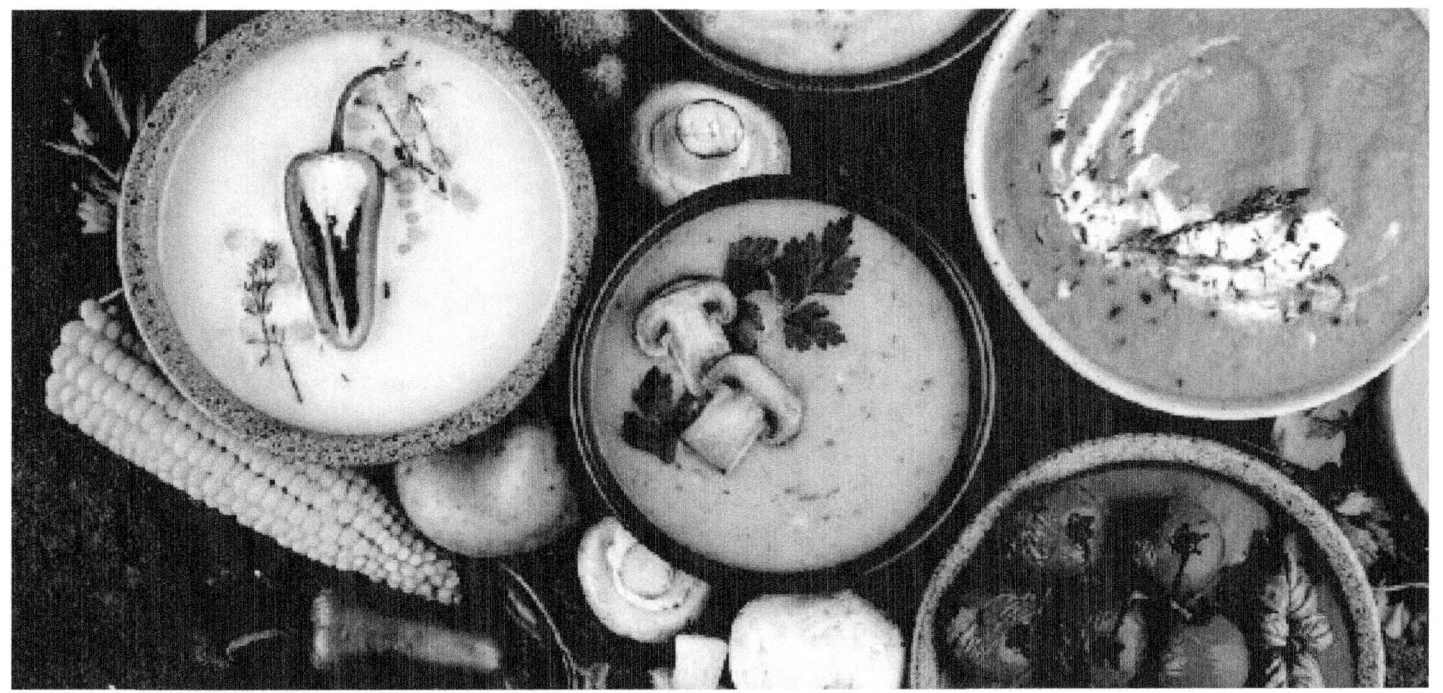

CHAPTER 5
SOUPS AND STEWS

"A warm bowl of immense healing - each delicious spoonful, a conscious step toward wellness."

Soups and stews are perfect vehicles for delivering anti-inflammatory ingredients in a delicious and nourishing way.

In this chapter, you'll find a variety of recipes rich in antioxidants, omega-3 fatty acids, and healing herbs that are known to combat inflammation.

These dishes are designed to be both comforting and healing, featuring ingredients that support a balanced, anti-inflammatory lifestyle.

TIPS:

- **LOW AND SLOW COOKING:** Cooking soups and stews over a low heat for longer periods allows the flavors to melt together.

- **STORAGE:** Store soups in the refrigerator for up to 3–4 days. For longer storage, soups can be frozen for up to 3 months.

- **LOW SODIUM BROTH:** When buying store-bought broth for anti-inflammatory soups, choose low-sodium options without additives, preservatives, or added sugars. Opt for organic or "no added MSG" broths for a healthier choice.

CARROT AND CHICKEN SOUP

SF, GF, NF, DF

PREP TIME: 10 mins   **COOK TIME:** 20 mins   **SERVINGS:** 4

CALORIES: 230 | PROTEIN: 25G | CARBS: 15G | FAT: 9G | FIBER: 3G

- 1 lb (450g) chicken breasts
- 1 tbsp olive oil
- 1 onion, diced
- 2 cloves garlic, minced
- 1 tbsp fresh ginger, grated
- 1 tbsp turmeric powder
- 4 cups (1 liter) chicken broth
- 1 cup (120g) carrots, sliced
- 1 cup (120g) celery, sliced
- 1 cup (30g) spinach leaves
- Salt, pepper, and lemon juice to taste
- ¼ cup coconut milk (optional)

1. In a large pot, heat olive oil over medium heat (160°C / 320°F). Add diced onion and garlic, sauté until softened, about 3-4 minutes.
2. Stir in grated ginger and turmeric powder, cooking for another minute until fragrant. Add diced chicken and pour in chicken broth. Bring to a simmer and cook for 10 minutes until chicken is cooked through.
3. Remove the chicken, shred it, and return it to the pot. Add carrots, celery, and spinach. Cook until vegetables are tender, about 5-7 minutes.
4. Season with salt, pepper, and lemon juice to taste. Serve hot and drizzle coconut milk if desired.

SWEET POTATO & LENTIL STEW

VG, SF, GF, NF, V

PREP TIME: 10 mins   **COOK TIME:** 20 mins   **SERVINGS:** 4

CALORIES: 220 | PROTEIN: 12G | CARBS: 35G | FAT: 4G | FIBER: 8G

- 1 tbsp olive oil
- 1 onion, chopped
- 2 cloves garlic, minced
- 1 tbsp fresh ginger, grated
- 1 tsp turmeric powder
- 1 tsp cumin
- 1 tsp paprika
- 1 cup (200g) dried lentils, rinsed
- 2 cups (500ml) vegetable broth
- 2 cups (300g) sweet potatoes, cubed
- ¼ cup diced tomatoes
- 1 cup (120g) kale, chopped
- Salt, pepper, and lemon juice to taste

1. Heat olive oil in a large pot over medium heat. Add diced onion, garlic, and ginger; cook for 3-4 minutes until softened.
2. Stir in rinsed lentils and cook for 1 minute.
3. Add sweet potatoes, diced tomatoes, vegetable broth, cumin, paprika, and turmeric.
4. Bring to a boil, then reduce heat to a simmer. Cook for 15-20 minutes, or until lentils and sweet potatoes are tender.
5. Stir in kale and cook for another 2-3 minutes until wilted.
6. Season with salt and pepper to taste, then serve hot.

GREEN DETOX SOUP

VG, GF, SF, NF, V

PREP TIME: 10 mins   **COOK TIME:** 20 mins   **SERVINGS:** 4

CALORIES: 180 | PROTEIN: 6G | CARBS: 30G | FAT: 4G | FIBER: 8G

- 1 tbsp olive oil
- 1 onion, diced
- 2 cloves garlic, minced
- 4 cups (960ml) vegetable broth
- 2 cups (120g) spinach leaves
- 2 cups (200g) broccoli florets
- 1 cup (100g) zucchini, diced
- ½ cup (60g) green peas (fresh or frozen)
- 1 tsp ground turmeric
- Salt and pepper to taste
- 1 tbsp lemon juice (optional)

1. Heat olive oil in a large pot over medium heat.
2. Sauté diced onion and garlic until softened, about 3-4 minutes.
3. Add vegetable broth, spinach, broccoli, zucchini, and green peas. Bring to a boil.
4. Reduce heat and simmer for 15 minutes, or until vegetables are tender.
5. Blend the soup with an immersion blender until smooth.
6. Stir in lemon juice if using, and season with salt, pepper, and turmeric to taste.
7. Serve warm.

SPICY TOMATO AND BASIL SOUP

VG, GF, SF, NF, V

PREP TIME: 5 mins **COOK TIME:** 25 mins **SERVINGS:** 4

CALORIES: 150 | PROTEIN: 3G | CARBS: 20G | FAT: 6G | FIBER: 5G

- 1 tbsp olive oil
- 1 onion, diced
- 3 cloves garlic, minced
- 5 large tomatoes, chopped
- 3 cups (720ml) vegetable broth
- ½ cup fresh basil leaves
- Salt and pepper to taste
- ½ tsp smoked paprika (optional)

1. Heat olive oil in a large pot over medium heat.
2. Sauté diced onion and garlic for 3-4 minutes until softened.
3. Add chopped tomatoes and vegetable broth. Bring to a boil, then reduce heat and simmer for 15-20 minutes.
4. Add fresh basil leaves and blend the soup with an immersion blender until smooth.
5. Season with salt, pepper, and smoked paprika if desired.
6. Serve hot and enjoy!

QUICK BROCCOLI SOUP

VG, GF, NF, SF, V
(IF USING SOY FREE VERSION)

PREP TIME: 5 mins **COOK TIME:** 25 mins **SERVINGS:** 4

CALORIES: 180 | PROTEIN: 5G | CARBS: 30G | FAT: 6G | FIBER: 6G

- 1 tbsp olive oil
- 1 onion, chopped
- 2 cloves garlic, minced
- 4 cups (400g) broccoli florets
- 4 cups (1 liter) vegetable broth
- ½ cup (125ml) coconut milk (optional)
- Salt and pepper to taste

1. Heat olive oil in a pot over medium heat.
2. Sauté onion and garlic until softened, about 5 minutes.
3. Add broccoli and vegetable broth, bring to a boil.
4. Reduce heat and simmer for 15-20 minutes, until broccoli is tender.
5. Blend the soup using an immersion blender until smooth.
6. Stir in coconut milk (if using) and season with salt and pepper.

MISO AND TOFU SOUP

VG, GF, DF, V

PREP TIME: 10 mins **COOK TIME:** 15 mins **SERVINGS:** 4

CALORIES: 180 | CARBS: 10G | FAT: 12G | PROTEIN: 12G | FIBER: 2G

- 1 tbsp sesame oil
- 1 medium onion, chopped
- 2 garlic cloves, minced
- 1 tsp grated fresh ginger
- 750 ml vegetable stock
- 3 tbsp miso paste
- 200 g firm tofu, cubed
- 1 tsp soy sauce (or tamari for GF)
- ½ tsp chili flakes
- Chopped green onions for garnish

1. Heat sesame oil in a pot. Sauté onion, garlic, and ginger until softened.
2. Add vegetable stock and bring to a simmer.
3. Stir in miso paste and soy sauce, then add tofu and chili flakes. Simmer for 5 minutes.
4. Season with salt and pepper. Garnish with green onions before serving.

CURRIED PARSNIP AND APPLE SOUP

VG, GF, DF, SF, NF, V

PREP TIME: 10 mins **COOK TIME:** 20 mins **SERVINGS:** 4

CALORIES: 180 | CARBS: 30G | FAT: 5G | PROTEIN: 2G | FIBER: 6G

- 500 g parsnips, peeled and chopped
- 1 apple, peeled and chopped
- 1 medium onion, chopped
- 1 tbsp olive oil
- 1 tsp curry powder
- ½ tsp ground ginger
- 750 ml vegetable stock
- Salt and pepper to taste
- Coconut cream (optional, for garnish)

1. Heat olive oil in a pot over medium heat. Sauté onion until softened.
2. Add curry powder and ginger. Stir for 1 minute.
3. Add parsnips, apple, and vegetable stock. Simmer for 15 minutes until tender.
4. Blend until smooth. Season with salt and pepper. Garnish with coconut cream if desired.

PUMPKIN AND CORN SOUP

VG, GF, DF, SF, NF, V

PREP TIME: 10 mins **COOK TIME:** 20 mins **SERVINGS:** 4

CALORIES: 180 | CARBS: 28G | FAT: 5G | PROTEIN: 4G | FIBER: 6G

- 400 g pumpkin, peeled and cubed
- 200 g sweet corn kernels (fresh or frozen)
- 1 medium onion, chopped
- 2 garlic cloves, minced
- 1 tbsp olive oil
- ½ tsp smoked paprika
- ½ tsp ground cumin
- 1 L vegetable stock
- Salt and pepper to taste
- 2 tbsp coconut milk
- Fresh parsley or cilantro for garnish

1. Heat olive oil in a large pot over medium heat. Sauté onion and garlic for 3–4 minutes until fragrant.
2. Add pumpkin cubes and cook for 5 minutes, stirring occasionally.
3. Stir in smoked paprika, cumin, salt, and pepper. Cook for 1 minute.
4. Add vegetable stock and bring to a boil. Reduce heat and simmer for 10–12 minutes until pumpkin is tender.
5. Stir in corn and cook for another 2–3 minutes.
6. Blend the soup partially with an immersion blender, leaving some chunks for texture.
7. Stir in coconut milk (if using) and adjust seasoning as needed.
8. Garnish with parsley or cilantro before serving.

OKRA AND TOMATO STEW

GF, VG, NF, V

PREP TIME: 10 mins **COOK TIME:** 20 mins **SERVINGS:** 4

CALORIES: 170 | PROTEIN: 3G | CARBS: 15G | FAT: 9G | FIBER: 5G

- 500g (18 oz) fresh or frozen okra
- 1 medium onion, finely chopped
- 2 medium tomatoes, peeled and chopped
- 1 tbsp tomato paste
- 2 tbsp olive oil
- 1 tbsp lemon juice
- 1 cup (250 ml) vegetable stock or water
- ½ tsp salt
- ½ tsp black pepper
- ½ tsp paprika

1. Heat olive oil in a large pot over medium heat. Add the chopped onion and sauté until softened, about 2-3 minutes.
2. Stir in the tomato paste and cook for 1 minute, releasing its flavor.
3. Add the chopped tomatoes and cook for another 3-4 minutes until softened.
4. Add the okra, lemon juice, vegetable stock, salt, pepper, and paprika. Mix well.
5. Bring the mixture to a gentle boil, then lower the heat. Cover and simmer for 15 minutes, stirring occasionally, until the okra is tender.
6. Serve warm, garnished with fresh parsley if desired, alongside bread or rice.

BUTTERNUT SQUASH & CHICKPEA SOUP

VG, GF, SF, NF, V

PREP TIME: 10 mins **COOK TIME:** 20 mins **SERVINGS:** 4

CALORIES: 250 | PROTEIN: 8G | CARBS: 40G | FAT: 6G | FIBER: 10G

- 1 tbsp olive oil
- 1 onion, diced
- 2 cloves garlic, minced
- 1 tbsp fresh ginger, grated
- 1 tsp turmeric powder
- 1 tsp paprika
- 1 can (400g) chickpeas, drained
- 4 cups (1 liter) vegetable broth
- 3 cups (400g) butternut squash, cubed
- 1 tsp cumin
- 1 cup (30g) fresh basil leaves
- Salt, pepper, and lemon juice to taste
- ¼ cup coconut milk (optional for creaminess)

1. Heat olive oil in a large pot over medium heat.
2. Add diced onion and garlic; sauté for 3-4 minutes until softened.
3. Add cubed butternut squash, chickpeas, vegetable broth, cumin, and turmeric.
4. Bring the mixture to a boil, then reduce heat and simmer for 15-20 minutes, or until the squash is tender.
5. Use an immersion blender to blend the soup until smooth. Stir in coconut milk if using.
6. Season with salt and pepper to taste, then serve warm.

QUICK ANTI-INFLAMMATORY VEGETABLE BROTH WITH NOODLES

VG, SF, GF, DF, V
PREP TIME: 5 mins **COOK TIME:** 25 mins **SERVINGS:** 4
CALORIES: 150 | PROTEIN: 12G | CARBS: 4G | FAT: 8G | FIBER: 1G

- 1 tbsp olive oil
- 1 onion, quartered
- 2 cloves garlic, smashed
- 1 tbsp fresh ginger, sliced
- 100g rice noodles (gluten-free if needed)
- 1 tsp ground turmeric
- 4 cups water or vegetable broth
- 1 bay leaf
- 1 celery stalk, roughly chopped
- ½ tsp black peppercorns
- Salt to taste
- ¼ tsp cayenne pepper
- 2 medium carrots, roughly chopped
- Fresh herbs (like parsley or cilantro) for garnish

1. Heat olive oil in a pot over medium heat.
2. Sauté onion, garlic, ginger, and turmeric for 3-4 minutes until fragrant.
3. Add carrots, celery, water or vegetable broth, bay leaf, and black peppercorns. Bring to a boil.
4. Reduce heat and simmer for 15-20 minutes, partially covered.
5. Add noodles and cook according to package (typically 5-7 minutes).
6. Strain the broth if desired, season with salt and cayenne pepper, and remove the bay leaf.
7. Serve warm with noodles and garnish with fresh herbs.

QUICK BEEF AND POTATO STEW

GF, NF
PREP TIME: 10 mins **COOK TIME:** 20 mins **SERVINGS:** 4
CALORIES: 340 | PROTEIN: 20G | CARBS: 23G | FAT: 14G | FIBER: 3G

- 400g (14 oz) beef strips or quick-cooking stew meat
- 2 medium potatoes, peeled and diced
- 2 medium carrots, thinly sliced
- 1 medium onion, finely chopped
- 2 garlic cloves, minced
- 2 tbsp olive oil
- 2 cups (500 ml) beef stock
- 1 cup (250g) tomato puree
- 1 tsp smoked paprika
- 1 tsp dried thyme
- ½ tsp salt
- ½ tsp black pepper

1. Heat olive oil in a large pot over medium-high heat. Sear the beef strips for 2-3 minutes until browned. Remove and set aside.
2. In the same pot, sauté the onion and garlic for 2 minutes until soft.
3. Add smoked paprika, thyme, and tomato puree. Cook for 1 minute, stirring.
4. Pour in the beef stock and bring to a boil. Add the diced potatoes and carrots, then simmer on medium heat for 12-15 minutes until tender.
5. Return the beef to the pot, season with salt and pepper, and cook for 3 more minutes to heat through.
6. Serve hot, garnished with fresh parsley if desired.

MOROCCAN CHICKEN AND APRICOT STEW

GF, DF, SF, NF
PREP TIME: 5 mins
COOK TIME: 25 mins **SERVINGS:** 4
CALORIES: 310 | CARBS: 22G | FAT: 18G | PROTEIN: 28G | FIBER: 6G

- 500 g chicken thighs, boneless and skinless
- 1 tbsp olive oil
- 1 medium onion, chopped
- 2 garlic cloves, minced
- 1/2 cup dried apricots, chopped
- 750 ml chicken stock
- 1 tsp ground cumin
- 1/2 tsp cinnamon
- Salt and pepper to taste

1. Heat olive oil in a large pot. Brown chicken thighs and set aside.
2. In the same pot, sauté onion and garlic until softened.
3. Add apricots, chicken stock, cumin, and cinnamon.
4. Simmer for 20-25 minutes.
5. Season with salt and pepper before serving.

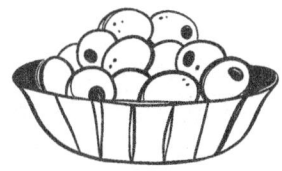

MINESTRONE SOUP

VG, DF, SF, NF, GF (OPTIONAL), V
PREP TIME: 10 mins **COOK TIME:** 20 mins **SERVINGS:** 4
CALORIES: 230 | CARBS: 40G | FAT: 6G | PROTEIN: 9G | FIBER: 8G

- 100 g dry pasta (small shapes like elbow or ditalini)
- 1 tbsp olive oil
- 1 medium onion, chopped
- 2 carrots, diced
- 2 celery stalks, diced
- 2 cloves garlic, minced
- 1 zucchini, diced
- 1 can (400 g) diced tomatoes
- 1 can (400 g) cannellini beans, drained and rinsed
- 1.5 L vegetable stock
- 1 tsp dried oregano
- ½ tsp dried thyme
- Salt and pepper to taste
- 2 cups spinach, chopped
- Fresh basil for garnish

1. Heat olive oil in a large pot over medium heat. Sauté onion, carrots, and celery for 5 minutes until softened.
2. Add garlic and zucchini and cook for 2 more minutes. Stir in oregano, thyme, salt, and pepper.
3. Pour in diced tomatoes, cannellini beans, and vegetable stock. Bring to a boil. Add pasta and cook for 8–10 minutes, or until pasta is tender.
4. Stir in spinach and cook for another 2 minutes. Taste and adjust seasoning with salt and pepper.
5. Garnish with fresh basil before serving.

SPANISH CHORIZO AND BEAN STEW

GF
PREP TIME: 10 mins **COOK TIME:** 20 mins **SERVINGS:** 4
CALORIES: 320 | PROTEIN: 15G | CARBS: 28G | FAT: 16G | FIBER: 7G

- 200g (7 oz) chorizo sausage, sliced
- 2 cups (400g) cooked white or pinto beans
- 1 medium potato, peeled and cubed
- 1 medium carrot, sliced
- 1 small onion, finely chopped
- 2 garlic cloves, minced
- 1 tbsp olive oil
- 2 cups (500 ml) vegetable or chicken stock
- 1 cup (250g) tomato puree
- 1 tsp smoked paprika
- 1 bay leaf
- 1 tsp salt
- 1 tsp black pepper
- Fresh parsley for garnish

1. Heat olive oil in a large pot over medium heat. Add the sliced chorizo and cook for 3-4 minutes until it releases its oils. Remove and set aside.
2. In the same pot, sauté the onion and garlic for 2-3 minutes until fragrant.
3. Stir in the smoked paprika, bay leaf, and tomato puree. Cook for 2 minutes to enhance the flavors.
4. Add the potato, carrot, and cooked beans. Pour in the stock, then season with salt and pepper. Bring to a boil.
5. Reduce the heat and simmer for 15 minutes, until the vegetables are tender.
6. Return the chorizo to the pot and simmer for another 5 minutes to heat through.
7. Serve warm, garnished with fresh parsley.

CHICKPEA AND TOMATO STEW

VG, GF, DF, NF, V
PREP TIME: 5 mins
COOK TIME: 25 mins **SERVINGS:** 4
CALORIES: 220 | CARBS: 40G | FAT: 7G | PROTEIN: 10G | FIBER: 10G

- 1 tbsp olive oil
- 1 medium onion, chopped
- 2 garlic cloves, minced
- 1 can (400g) chickpeas, drained and rinsed
- 400 g canned tomatoes
- 750 ml vegetable stock
- 1 tsp ground cumin
- 1/2 tsp paprika
- Salt and pepper to taste

1. Heat olive oil in a large pot. Sauté onion and garlic until softened.
2. Add chickpeas, tomatoes, vegetable stock, cumin, and paprika.
3. Simmer for 25 minutes.
4. Season with salt and pepper before serving.

ZESTY BLACK BEAN SOUP

VG, GF, DF, SF, NF, V

PREP TIME: 10 mins **COOK TIME:** 20 mins **SERVINGS:** 4

CALORIES: 220 | CARBS: 38G | FAT: 5G | PROTEIN: 8G | FIBER: 10G

- 1 tbsp olive oil
- 1 medium onion, chopped
- 2 garlic cloves, minced
- 1 red bell pepper, diced
- 1 tsp ground cumin
- ½ tsp smoked paprika
- ¼ tsp chili powder
- 400 g canned black beans, rinsed and drained
- 300 g canned corn, drained
- 750 ml vegetable stock
- Juice of 1 lime
- Fresh cilantro for garnish

1. Heat olive oil in a pot. Sauté onion, garlic, and bell pepper until softened. Add cumin, paprika, and chili powder. Stir for 1 minute.
2. Add black beans, corn, and vegetable stock. Simmer for 15 minutes.
3. Stir in lime juice and season with salt and pepper. Garnish with cilantro before serving.

SPICY LEMONGRASS CHICKEN SOUP

GF, DF, SF, NF

PREP TIME: 10 mins **COOK TIME:** 20 mins **SERVINGS:** 4

CALORIES: 230 | CARBS: 5G | FAT: 12G | PROTEIN: 25G | FIBER: 1G

- 1 tbsp olive oil
- 1 medium onion, chopped
- 2 garlic cloves, minced
- 1 stalk lemongrass, bruised
- 300 g chicken breast, thinly sliced
- 500 ml chicken stock
- 1 tbsp fish sauce (optional)
- ½ tsp chili flakes
- 1 tbsp lime juice
- Fresh cilantro for garnish

1. Heat olive oil in a pot. Sauté onion and garlic until softened.
2. Add lemongrass and chicken, cooking until chicken is browned.
3. Pour in chicken stock, fish sauce, and chili flakes. Simmer for 15 minutes.
4. Stir in lime juice and season with salt and pepper. Garnish with cilantro before serving.

TURKEY AND VEGETABLE STEW

GF, DF, SF, NF

PREP TIME: 5 mins **COOK TIME:** 25 mins **SERVINGS:** 4

CALORIES: 280 | CARBS: 20G | FAT: 15G | PROTEIN: 28G | FIBER: 5G

- 500 g ground turkey
- 1 tbsp olive oil
- 1 medium onion, chopped
- 2 garlic cloves, minced
- 1 bell pepper, chopped
- 1 zucchini, chopped
- 750 ml chicken stock
- 1 tsp dried oregano
- Salt and pepper to taste

1. Heat olive oil in a large pot. Brown ground turkey and set aside.
2. In the same pot, sauté onion and garlic until softened.
3. Add bell pepper, zucchini, chicken stock, and oregano. Simmer for 20 minutes.
4. Add turkey back in and simmer for another 5 minutes.
5. Season with salt and pepper before serving.

WHITE FISH STEW

GF, DF, NF

PREP TIME: 5 mins **COOK TIME:** 25 mins **SERVINGS:** 4

CALORIES: 230 | CARBS: 18G | FAT: 8G | PROTEIN: 28G | FIBER: 4G

- 500 g white fish fillets (such as cod or tilapia), cut into chunks
- 1 tbsp olive oil
- 1 medium onion, chopped
- 2 garlic cloves, minced
- 400 g canned diced tomatoes
- 750 ml fish stock
- 1 tsp dried basil
- Salt and pepper to taste

1. Heat olive oil in a large pot. Sauté onion and garlic until softened.
2. Add diced tomatoes, fish stock, and basil. Bring to a simmer.
3. Add fish chunks and cook for 15-20 minutes until fish is tender.
4. Season with salt and pepper before serving.

LAMB AND EGGPLANT STEW

GF, DF, SF, NF

PREP TIME: 5 mins **COOK TIME:** 25 mins **SERVINGS:** 4

CALORIES: 320 | CARBS: 20G | FAT: 22G | PROTEIN: 28G | FIBER: 6G

- 500 g lamb stew chunks
- 1 tbsp olive oil
- 1 medium onion, chopped
- 2 garlic cloves, minced
- 1 medium eggplant, cubed
- 500 ml lamb stock
- 1 tsp cumin
- 1 tsp paprika
- Salt and pepper to taste

1. Heat olive oil in a large pot. Brown lamb chunks and set aside.
2. In the same pot, sauté onion and garlic until softened.
3. Add eggplant, lamb stock, cumin, and paprika. Simmer for 20 minutes.
4. Season with salt and pepper before serving.

CAULIFLOWER AND LEEK SOUP

VG, GF, NF, SF, V

PREP TIME: 5 mins **COOK TIME:** 25 mins **SERVINGS:** 4

CALORIES: 190 | PROTEIN: 4G | CARBS: 30G | FAT: 7G | FIBER: 6G

- 1 tbsp olive oil
- 1 leek, chopped
- 2 cloves garlic, minced
- 4 cups (1 liter) vegetable broth
- 4 cups (400g) cauliflower florets
- Salt and pepper to taste

1. Heat olive oil in a pot over medium heat.
2. Sauté leek and garlic for 5 minutes until tender.
3. Add cauliflower and vegetable broth, and bring to a boil.
4. Reduce heat and simmer for 20 minutes until cauliflower is soft.
5. Blend the soup until smooth, season with salt and pepper, and serve warm.

CHICKEN AND VEGETABLE STEW WITH MUSHROOMS

GF, NF, DF (OPTIONAL)

PREP TIME: 10 mins **COOK TIME:** 20 mins **SERVINGS:** 4

CALORIES: 310 | PROTEIN: 28G | CARBS: 15G | FAT: 12G | FIBER: 3G

- 400g (14 oz) boneless chicken breast or thighs, cubed
- 1 cup (150g) diced butternut squash
- 1 cup (150g) mushrooms, quartered
- 1 medium onion, finely chopped
- 2 garlic cloves, minced
- 1 ½ tbsp olive oil
- 1 ½ cups (375 ml) chicken stock
- ½ cup (125 ml) coconut cream or dairy-free cream (use heavy cream if not dairy-free)
- 1 tsp dried thyme
- ½ tsp smoked paprika
- ½ tsp salt
- ¼ tsp black pepper
- Fresh thyme sprigs for garnish (optional)

1. Heat olive oil in a large pot over medium-high heat. Add the chicken and cook for 4 minutes until lightly browned. Remove and set aside.
2. In the same pot, sauté the onion and garlic for 2 minutes until fragrant. Add the butternut squash and mushrooms. Cook for 3 minutes, stirring occasionally.
3. Stir in thyme, smoked paprika, and chicken stock. Bring to a boil, then lower the heat to medium. Cover and simmer for 10 minutes until the squash is tender.
4. Return the chicken to the pot and pour in the coconut cream or heavy cream. Simmer for an additional 3 minutes, stirring to combine.
5. Season with salt and pepper to taste. Serve hot, garnished with fresh thyme if desired.

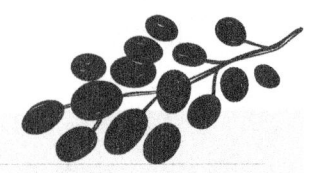

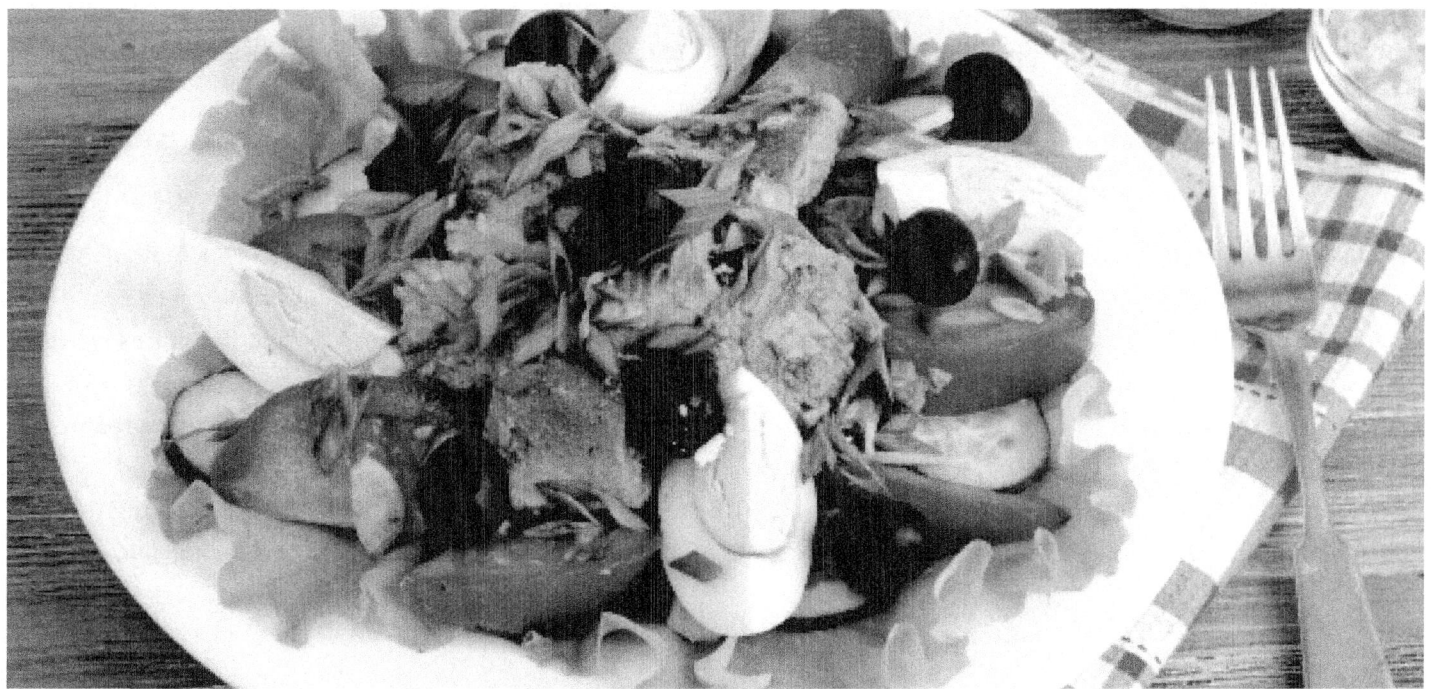

CHAPTER 6

SALADS

"Color your plate with a rainbow - calm your body and reset your immunity."

Creating a salad with vibrant vegetables, leafy greens, and antioxidant-rich fruits can be a delicious way to support your body's fight against inflammation.

Ingredients such as spinach, kale, berries, avocados, and nuts provide essential nutrients that help reduce inflammation naturally.

To elevate the anti-inflammatory properties, consider adding flavorful extras like olive oil, turmeric, or ginger for a powerful health boost.

TIPS:

- **HEALTHY FATS ARE KEY:** Add walnuts, flaxseeds, or avocados for a boost of omega-3s.

- **STORAGE:** Store salads in an airtight container with a paper towel on top to absorb moisture. Keep dressing separate. Salads stay fresh for 2-3 days.

SPINACH AND BERRIES SALAD

GF, V, DF, VG

PREP TIME: 10 mins **COOK TIME:** 0 min **SERVINGS:** 4

CALORIES: 180 | PROTEIN: 4G | CARBS: 16G | FAT: 12G | FIBER: 4G

- 4 cups fresh spinach
- 1 cup mixed berries (strawberries, blueberries, raspberries)
- ¼ cup walnuts, chopped (toast lightly for more flavor)
- ¼ cup crumbled feta (optional)
- 1 small red onion, thinly sliced
- ¼ cup pomegranate seeds
- 1 tbsp fresh mint leaves, chopped
- ¼ cup balsamic vinaigrette
- 1 tsp Dijon mustard
- Salt and pepper to taste
- Blanched asparagus (optional)

1. Toast the walnuts in a dry pan over medium heat for 2-3 minutes until they're fragrant. Set aside to cool.
2. In a small bowl, whisk together the balsamic vinaigrette, Dijon mustard, salt, and pepper.
3. In a large bowl, combine the spinach, berries, walnuts, red onion, pomegranate seeds, and mint.
4. Drizzle with the balsamic-Dijon dressing and gently toss to mix.
5. Sprinkle with crumbled feta, if using, and serve immediately.

TUNA AND EGG SALAD WITH OLIVES

GF, SF, DF, NF

PREP TIME: 10 mins **COOK TIME:** 0 min **SERVINGS:** 1

CALORIES: 376 | PROTEIN: 21G | CARBS: 26G | FAT: 16G | FIBER: 6G

- 1 (5-ounce) can chunk light tuna in water, drained
- 5-6 black olives, whole or sliced
- 1 boiled egg, halved or quartered
- 1 medium tomato, sliced into wedges
- 1 small cucumber, thinly sliced
- A handful of fresh lettuce leaves
- 1-2 tbsp fresh green onions, chopped
- 1 ½ tbsp olive oil
- 1 tbsp lemon juice
- Salt and black pepper to taste

1. Arrange the lettuce leaves on a plate, creating a base. Add the sliced tomatoes and cucumber on top.
2. Place the drained tuna chunks in the center of the salad. Surround with boiled egg quarters and olives.
3. In a small bowl, whisk together olive oil, lemon juice, salt, and black pepper and drizzle the dressing over the salad.
4. Sprinkle chopped green onions on top for added flavor.

ZUCCHINI AND CORN SALAD

VG, GF, DF, SF, NF, V

PREP TIME: 10 mins **COOK TIME:** 10 mins **SERVINGS:** 4

CALORIES: 150 | CARBS: 22G | FAT: 7G | PROTEIN: 3G | FIBER: 5G

- 2 medium zucchinis, thinly sliced
- 1 cup fresh corn kernels
- ½ red bell pepper, chopped
- 2 tbsp olive oil
- 1 tbsp lemon juice
- 1 tsp ground cumin
- Salt and pepper to taste

1. Heat 1 tbsp olive oil in a pan and sauté the zucchini slices and corn for 5-10 minutes until tender.
2. Transfer to a bowl and add the bell pepper.
3. Drizzle with olive oil and lemon juice, then sprinkle cumin, salt, and pepper.
4. Toss to combine and serve.

CRUNCHY CABBAGE & PUMPKIN SEED SLAW

VG, GF, DF, SF, V

PREP TIME: 10 mins **COOK TIME:** 0 min **SERVINGS:** 4

CALORIES: 160 | CARBS: 12G | FAT: 12G | PROTEIN: 4G | FIBER: 6G

- 2 cups shredded cabbage
- ¼ cup pumpkin seeds
- 1 small carrot, grated
- 1 tbsp apple cider vinegar
- 1 tbsp olive oil
- 1 tsp honey
- Salt and pepper to taste

1. In a large bowl, combine shredded cabbage, carrot, and pumpkin seeds.
2. In a small bowl, whisk together apple cider vinegar, olive oil, honey, salt, and pepper.
3. Pour dressing over cabbage mixture and toss to coat.
4. Serve chilled or at room temperature.

CITRUS BLACK BEAN QUINOA SALAD

GF, VG, SF, DF, V

PREP TIME: 15 mins **COOK TIME:** 0 min **SERVINGS:** 4

CALORIES: 230 | PROTEIN: 8G | CARBS: 35G | FAT: 5G | FIBER: 8G

- 1 cup cooked quinoa
- 1 cup black beans, rinsed and drained
- 1 cup diced bell peppers
- ½ cup cherry tomatoes, halved
- ¼ cup chopped cilantro
- ½ avocado
- 1 tsp pumpkin seeds
- Juice of 1 lime
- 2 tbsp olive oil
- Salt and pepper to taste

1. In a bowl, combine quinoa, black beans, bell peppers, tomatoes, avocado, and cilantro.
2. In a small bowl, whisk together lime juice, olive oil, salt, and pepper. Sprinkle pumpkin seeds.
3. Pour the dressing over the salad and toss to combine.

PEAR AND WALNUT SALAD

VG, GF, DF, SF, V

PREP TIME: 10 mins **COOK TIME:** 0 min **SERVINGS:** 4

CALORIES: 220 | CARBS: 23G | FAT: 15G | PROTEIN: 4G | FIBER: 6G

- 2 ripe pears, sliced
- ¼ cup walnuts, toasted
- 2 cups mixed greens (arugula, spinach, or lettuce)
- ¼ cup crumbled blue cheese (optional)
- 1 tbsp olive oil
- 1 tbsp balsamic vinegar
- Salt and pepper to taste

1. In a large bowl, combine pears, toasted walnuts, and mixed greens.
2. Drizzle with olive oil and balsamic vinegar.
3. Sprinkle with blue cheese (if using) and season with salt and pepper.
4. Toss gently and serve.

BEETROOT AND BLACKBERRY SALAD WITH TOFU AND SEEDS

VG, GF, SF, DF, V

PREP TIME: 15 mins **COOK TIME:** 0 min **SERVINGS:** 1

CALORIES: 320 | PROTEIN: 18G | CARBS: 24G | FAT: 14G | FIBER: 6G

- 1 medium beetroot, cooked and diced into cubes
- ½ cup fresh blackberries
- 100g firm tofu, cubed (can be lightly grilled for texture)
- 1 tbsp pine nuts or sunflower seeds, toasted
- 1 tbsp fresh parsley or cilantro, chopped
- 1 tbsp olive oil
- 1 tbsp lemon juice
- ½ tsp maple syrup (optional, for sweetness)
- A pinch of salt and black pepper

1. Add diced beetroot, blackberries, and tofu cubes to a bowl.
2. Sprinkle the toasted pine nuts or sunflower seeds over the salad.
3. Whisk together olive oil, lemon juice, maple syrup (if using), salt, and pepper in a small bowl. Drizzle the dressing over the salad.
4. Finish with a sprinkle of fresh parsley or cilantro for an herby touch.

CHICKEN, BRUSSELS SPROUTS & MUSHROOM SALAD

GF, SF, DF, NF

PREP TIME: 15 mins **COOK TIME:** 0 min **SERVINGS:** 4

CALORIES: 432 | PROTEIN: 24G | CARBS: 15G | FAT: 31G | FIBER: 5G

- 6 tbsp olive oil
- 3 tbsp red-wine vinegar
- 1 ½ tbsp minced shallot
- 2 tsp chopped fresh thyme
- ½ tsp ground pepper
- 12 ounces shredded cooked chicken
- 4 cups shaved fresh cremini mushrooms
- 4 cups cooked Brussels sprouts
- 4 cups packed baby arugula
- 1 cup thinly sliced celery (diagonally)

1. In a large bowl, whisk together the olive oil, red-wine vinegar, minced shallot, fresh thyme, and ground pepper until well combined.
2. Add the shredded chicken, shaved mushrooms, Brussels sprouts, baby arugula, and celery to the bowl.
3. Toss everything together to coat the with the dressing. Serve and enjoy!

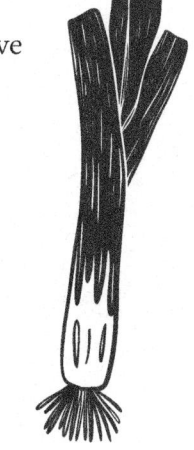

KALE, AVOCADO AND SWEET POTATO BOWL

GF, VG, DF, SF, V

PREP TIME: 15 mins   **COOK TIME:** 0 min   **SERVING:** 4

CALORIES: 220 | PROTEIN: 4G | CARBS: 14G | FAT: 8G | FIBER: 7G

- 4 cups kale, chopped
- 1 avocado, diced
- ¼ cup sweet potato
- ½ cup cooked quinoa
- 2 tbsp extra-virgin olive oil
- Juice of 1 lemon
- Salt and pepper to taste

1. Place the chopped kale in a large bowl and massage with the olive oil for 2-3 minutes until it softens and becomes tender.
2. Add the cooked quinoa, diced avocado, and sweet potato to the bowl with the kale.
3. Drizzle the salad with fresh lemon juice, season with salt and pepper, and toss gently to combine.
4. Serve immediately or refrigerate for up to 1 day for the flavors to meld.

MEDITERRANEAN CHICKPEA AND CUCUMBER SALAD

GF, VG, DF, SF, V

PREP TIME: 10 mins   **COOK TIME:** 0 min   **SERVINGS:** 4

CALORIES: 230 | PROTEIN: 9G | CARBS: 30G | FAT: 9G | FIBER: 14G

- 1 can (15 oz) chickpeas, drained and rinsed
- 1 cucumber, diced
- 1 red bell pepper, diced
- ¼ cup red onion, finely chopped
- 2 tbsp parsley, chopped
- 2 tbsp olive oil
- 1 tbsp red wine vinegar
- ½ tsp cumin powder
- Salt and pepper to taste

1. In a large bowl, combine the chickpeas, cucumber, bell pepper, red onion, and parsley.
2. In a small bowl, whisk together the olive oil, red wine vinegar, cumin, salt, and pepper.
3. Pour the dressing over the salad and toss well.
4. Serve immediately or refrigerate for up to 2 days.

ASIAN SESAME NOODLE SALAD

VG, DF, V

PREP TIME: 10 mins　　**COOK TIME:** 10 mins　　**SERVINGS:** 4

CALORIES: 220 | CARBS: 30G | FAT: 8G | PROTEIN: 4G | FIBER: 3G

- 200g rice noodles
- ½ cup shredded carrots
- ½ cup red bell pepper, thinly sliced
- ¼ cup green onions, chopped
- 2 tbsp sesame seeds, toasted
- 1 tbsp soy sauce (or tamari for GF)
- 1 tbsp sesame oil
- 1 tbsp rice vinegar

1. Cook rice noodles according to package and rinse under cold water.
2. Combine noodles, carrots, bell pepper, green onions, and sesame seeds in a bowl.
3. Drizzle with soy sauce, sesame oil, and rice vinegar. Toss to coat and serve.

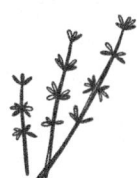

TURKEY COBB SALAD

GF, DF, SF

PREP TIME: 15 mins　　**COOK TIME:** 10 mins　　**SERVINGS:** 4

CALORIES: 280 | CARBS: 8G | FAT: 18G | PROTEIN: 21G | FIBER: 4G

- 200 g turkey breast, cooked and diced
- 4 cups romaine lettuce, chopped
- 100 g cherry tomatoes, halved
- 1 avocado, diced
- 2 boiled eggs, chopped
- 2 slices of cooked turkey bacon, crumbled
- 50 g blue cheese, crumbled
- 2 tbsp olive oil
- 1 tbsp red wine vinegar
- 1 tsp Dijon mustard
- Salt and pepper to taste

1. In a small bowl, whisk olive oil, red wine vinegar, Dijon mustard, salt, and pepper to make the dressing.
2. On a large platter, arrange romaine lettuce. Top with turkey, cherry tomatoes, avocado, eggs, turkey bacon, and blue cheese.
3. Drizzle the dressing over the salad and serve immediately.

GRILLED PEACH AND RICOTTA SALAD

VG, GF, NF, V

PREP TIME: 10 mins　　**COOK TIME:** 10 mins　　**SERVINGS:** 4

CALORIES: 190 | CARBS: 20G | FAT: 10G | PROTEIN: 6G | FIBER: 4G

- 4 peaches, halved and pitted
- ½ cup ricotta cheese
- 4 cups arugula
- ¼ cup almonds, toasted
- 1 tbsp honey
- 1 tbsp balsamic glaze
- 1 tbsp olive oil
- Salt and pepper to taste

1. Brush peaches with olive oil and grill for 3-4 minutes per side.
2. Arrange arugula on a plate, add grilled peaches, and dollop ricotta on top.
3. Sprinkle with almonds, drizzle with honey and balsamic glaze, and season with salt and pepper.

WATERCRESS SALAD

GF, DF, SF, NF

PREP TIME: 10 mins　　**COOK TIME:** 0 min　　**SERVINGS:** 4

CALORIES: 120 | CARBS: 3G | FAT: 10G | PROTEIN: 5G | FIBER: 1G

- 200 g watercress, washed
- 2 hard-boiled eggs, sliced
- 1 small red onion, thinly sliced
- 1 tbsp Dijon mustard
- 2 tbsp olive oil
- 1 tbsp apple cider vinegar
- Salt and pepper to taste

1. In a small bowl, whisk together Dijon mustard, olive oil, apple cider vinegar, salt, and pepper to make the dressing.
2. Arrange watercress on a serving plate. Top with hard-boiled egg slices and red onion.
3. Drizzle the dressing over the salad before serving.

THAI PAPAYA SALAD

VG, GF, DF, NF, V

PREP TIME: 15 mins **COOK TIME:** 0 min **SERVINGS:** 4

CALORIES: 120 | CARBS: 18G | FAT: 4G | PROTEIN: 3G | FIBER: 4G

- 300 g green papaya, peeled and shredded
- 100 g cherry tomatoes, halved
- 50 g green beans, trimmed and cut into 2-inch pieces
- 2 garlic cloves, minced
- 2 tbsp lime juice
- 1 tbsp fish sauce (or soy sauce for vegan)
- 1 tbsp palm sugar (or brown sugar)
- 1 red chili, finely chopped
- 2 tbsp roasted peanuts, crushed

1. In a small bowl, mix lime juice, fish sauce (or soy sauce), palm sugar, garlic, and chili to make the dressing.
2. In a large bowl, combine shredded papaya, cherry tomatoes, and green beans.
3. Pour the dressing over the salad and toss well.
4. Garnish with crushed roasted peanuts before serving.

THE ULTIMATE ARUGULA & FETA SALAD

GF, VG, DF, NF, V

PREP TIME: 10 mins **COOK TIME:** 0 min **SERVINGS:** 4

CALORIES: 250 | PROTEIN: 5G | CARBS: 18G | FAT: 5G | FIBER: 19G

- 4 cups fresh arugula
- ½ cup crumbled feta cheese (or a dairy-free alternative if needed)
- ½ cup pomegranate seeds
- ¼ cup walnuts, roughly chopped
- 2 tbsp capers (optional)
- ½ cup cherry tomatoes, quartered
- 3 tbsp extra-virgin olive oil
- 2 tbsp balsamic vinegar
- Salt and pepper to taste

1. In a large salad bowl, combine arugula, cherry tomatoes, pomegranate seeds, and walnuts.
2. Sprinkle the crumbled feta cheese and capers over the salad.
3. In a small bowl, whisk together the olive oil, balsamic vinegar, salt, and pepper.
4. Drizzle the dressing over the salad and toss gently to combine.
5. Serve immediately and enjoy!

MINTED LENTIL AND CUCUMBER SALAD

VG, GF, DF, SF, NF, V

PREP TIME: 10 mins **COOK TIME:** 15 mins **SERVINGS:** 4

CALORIES: 180 | CARBS: 28G | FAT: 6G | PROTEIN: 8G | FIBER: 8G

- 1 cup cooked green lentils
- 1 cucumber, diced
- ¼ cup fresh mint, chopped
- 1 tbsp olive oil
- 1 tbsp lemon juice
- Salt and pepper to taste

1. Combine cooked lentils, cucumber, and mint in a large bowl.
2. Drizzle with olive oil and lemon juice.
3. Season with salt and pepper and toss to combine.

EDAMAME AND SEAWEED SALAD

VG, GF, DF, V

PREP TIME: 10 mins **COOK TIME:** 0 min **SERVINGS:** 4

CALORIES: 130 | CARBS: 10G | FAT: 6G | PROTEIN: 9G | FIBER: 4G

- 1 cup cooked edamame
- ¼ cup wakame seaweed, soaked and drained
- 1 tbsp soy sauce (or tamari for GF)
- 1 tbsp rice vinegar
- 1 tsp sesame oil
- 1 tsp sesame seeds

1. Combine edamame and wakame in a bowl.
2. Drizzle with soy sauce, rice vinegar, and sesame oil.
3. Sprinkle with sesame seeds and toss to coat.

YOUR FREE GIFT
ANTI-INFLAMMATORY DIET BONUS BOOKS

Adopting the Anti-inflammatory diet is an integrated step-by-step process to heal the body, mind and spirit.

To help you embrace the Anti-inflammatory lifestyle where you can take small, practical steps daily to consciously choose nutrient-dense foods and manage the stresses of everyday living, here are three bonus eBooks specially designed to help you achieve a healthier life.

Bonus Book #1: 50 Powerful Anti-Inflammatory Ingredients Guidebook

This comprehensive guide dives into the heart of your anti-inflammatory journey by introducing 50 powerful ingredients that can *transform* your meals and health. Discover their science-backed benefits and how to use them in everyday meals.

Bonus Book #2: 45 Strategic Anti-inflammatory Dietary & Stress Management Practices

This bonus guide focuses on a matrix of *lifestyle, stress management and mindset practices* that will make your anti-inflammatory journey easier and more sustainable. Chronic inflammation isn't just influenced by diet - it's also affected by stress, emotions and daily habits.

Bonus Book #3: A Handbook of 100 Classic Anti-Inflammatory Recipes with Full Colored Pictures

Let this delightful recipe booklet be your go-to reference guide. Each recipe features *a special Health Perks section* and *a full colored photo* to help you identify the key elements of each food category so you can prep more meals with confidence.

TO GET INSTANT ACCESS GO TO:

https://heartbookspress.com/Anti-InflammatoryDietCookbook-FreeBonuses

You can also scan the QR Code below with your cell phone camera and tap on the link that pops up if you find that easier.

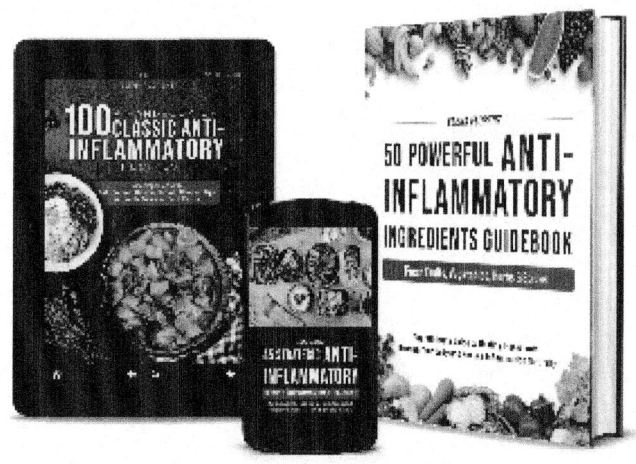

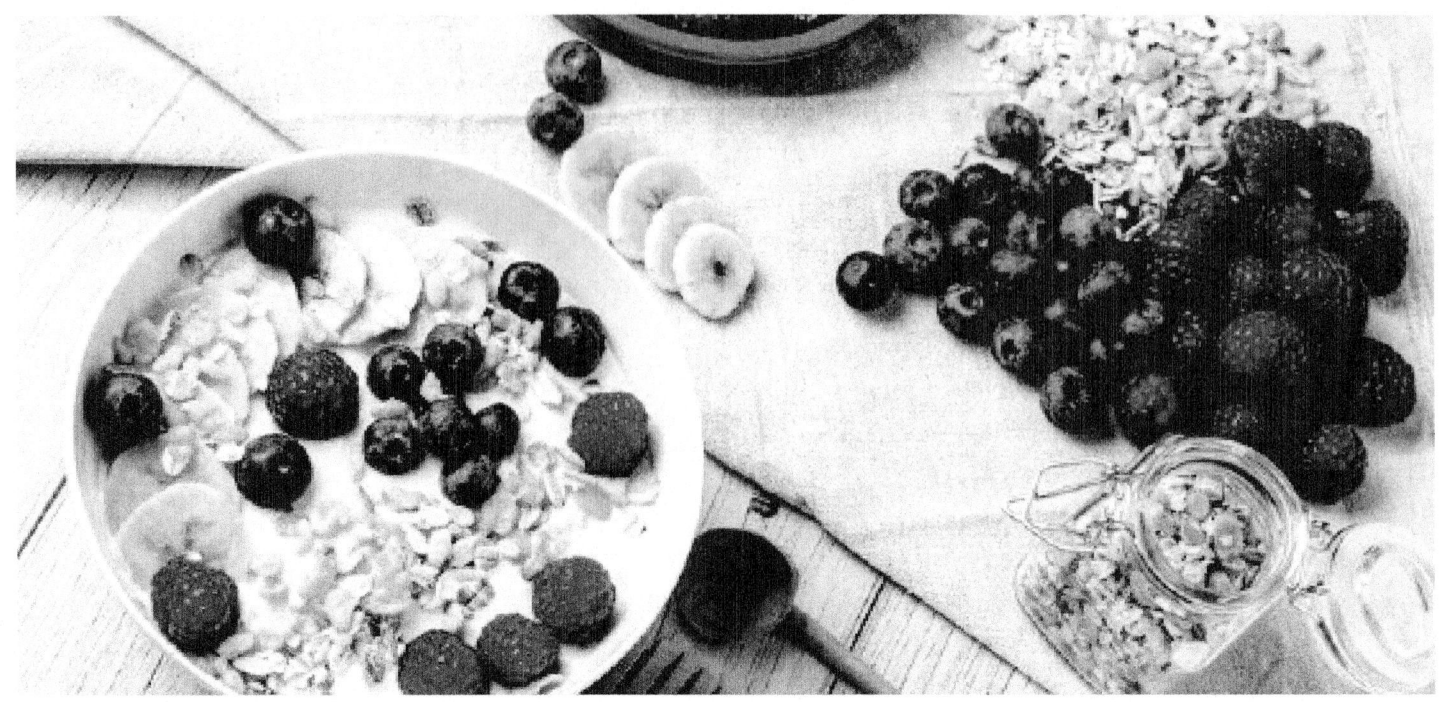

CHAPTER 7

BREAKFASTS

"Begin your day with bright foods that heal and nourish your body deeply."

The breakfasts focus on nutrient-dense foods that help reduce inflammation, which is linked to many chronic diseases like heart disease and arthritis.

Foods with omega-3 fatty acids, such as chia seeds or flaxseeds, is also common. These breakfasts are designed to stabilize blood sugar levels, boost energy, and promote overall wellness.

TIPS:

- **ANTIOXIDANTS:** Include foods rich in antioxidants (e.g. berries), fiber (e.g. oats), and omega-3s (e.g. flax or chia seeds) for a balanced anti-inflammatory meal.

- **STORAGE:** Overnight oats or chia puddings can be prepped in advance and stored in the fridge for up to 3 days. Smoothies can be frozen in single portions and thawed the night before for a quick grab-and-go option.

OATMEAL WITH FLAXSEEDS AND BLUEBERRIES

VG, GF (IF USING CERTIFIED OATS), SF, V

PREP TIME: 10 mins **COOK TIME:** 10 mins **SERVINGS:** 1

CALORIES: 250 | PROTEIN: 6G | CARBS: 45G | FAT: 7G | FIBER: 8G

- ½ cup rolled oats
- 1 cup water or almond milk
- 1 tbsp ground flaxseeds
- ½ cup fresh blueberries
- 1 tsp honey or maple syrup
- 1 tsp vanilla extract
- ½ tsp cinnamon
- 1 tbsp almond butter or peanut butter
- 1 tbsp chopped nuts (like walnuts or almonds for crunch)

1. In a saucepan, combine rolled oats with water or almond milk. Cook on medium heat for 5–10 minutes, stirring occasionally until the oats are creamy and cooked through.
2. Stir in ground flaxseeds, vanilla extract, and cinnamon, and let it sit for 1 minute to thicken.
3. Transfer the oatmeal to a bowl and top with fresh blueberries, a drizzle of honey or maple syrup, a dollop of almond or peanut butter, and chopped nuts.

QUICK CHIA SEEDS PUDDING WITH BERRIES

VG, GF, SF, V

PREP TIME: 5 mins **CHILLING TIME:** 20 mins **SERVINGS:** 4

CALORIES: 240 | PROTEIN: 6G | CARBS: 30G | FAT: 12G | FIBER: 10G

- 3 tbsp chia seeds
- 1 cup almond milk (or any dairy-free milk)
- 1 tsp maple syrup
- ½ cup mixed berries (fresh or frozen)
- 1 tbsp coconut flakes (unsweetened)
- 1 tsp vanilla extract
- ½ tsp cinnamon
- 1 tbsp nut butter
- 1 tbsp crushed nuts (such as walnuts or pistachios)
- Fresh mint leaves

1. In a mixing bowl, combine chia seeds, almond milk, maple syrup, vanilla extract, and cinnamon. Stir until well combined.
2. Let the mixture sit in the fridge for 15–20 minutes or overnight until it thickens to your desired consistency.
3. Before serving, top with mixed berries, coconut flakes, a dollop of nut butter, and crushed nuts for added texture.
4. Add fresh mint leaves for a pop of color and freshness.

CRISPY SWEET POTATO AND BLACK BEAN SKILLET

GF, DF, SF, NF, V

PREP TIME: 10 mins **COOK TIME:** 20 mins **SERVINGS:** 2

CALORIES: 270 | CARBS: 42G | FAT: 8G | PROTEIN: 7G | FIBER: 9G

- 1 medium sweet potato, diced
- ½ cup cooked black beans
- ¼ red onion, finely chopped
- 1 tbsp olive oil
- ½ tsp smoked paprika
- ¼ tsp ground cumin
- ¼ cup diced red bell pepper
- 1 tbsp chopped fresh cilantro
- 1 tbsp lime juice

1. Heat olive oil in a skillet and cook sweet potato until golden.
2. Add onion, bell pepper, black beans, paprika, and cumin. Cook for 5 more minutes.
3. Sprinkle with cilantro and lime juice before serving.

COCONUT YOGURT PARFAIT WITH BERRIES AND WALNUTS

VG, GF, SF, V

PREP TIME: 15 mins **COOK TIME:** 0 min **SERVINGS:** 1

CALORIES: 220 | PROTEIN: 4G | CARBS: 24G | FAT: 13G | FIBER: 5G

- ½ cup coconut yogurt
- ¼ cup mixed berries
- 1 tbsp chopped walnuts
- 1 tsp honey or maple syrup
- Dash of cinnamon
- 1 tbsp shredded coconut
- 1 tsp chia seeds
- Fresh mint leaves for garnish (optional)

1. Layer coconut yogurt, mixed berries, and walnuts in a bowl.
2. Drizzle with honey or maple syrup.
3. Sprinkle shredded coconut, chia seeds, and a dash of cinnamon for a flavorful twist.
4. Garnish with fresh mint leaves if desired.
5. Enjoy this parfait as a refreshing snack or light breakfast!

MISO GLAZED EGGPLANT AND RICE BREAKFAST BOWL

VG, GF, SF, V

PREP TIME: 10 mins   **COOK TIME:** 20 mins   **SERVINGS:** 2

CALORIES: 340 | CARBS: 55G | FAT: 9G | PROTEIN: 8G | FIBER: 7G

- 1 small eggplant, sliced
- 2 tbsp miso paste
- 1 tsp sesame oil
- 1 tsp honey (or maple syrup for vegan)
- 1 cup cooked brown rice
- ¼ cup shredded carrots
- 1 tsp sesame seeds

1. Roast eggplant brushed with miso, sesame oil, and honey until caramelized.
2. Serve on brown rice with shredded carrots and sesame seeds.

AVOCADO TOAST WITH TURMERIC & HEMP SEEDS

VG, GF, SF, DF, V

PREP TIME: 10 mins   **COOK TIME:** 0 min   **SERVINGS:** 1

CALORIES: 280 | PROTEIN: 7G | CARBS: 18G | FAT: 21G | FIBER: 8G

- 1 slice of whole grain/gluten-free bread (for gluten-free option)
- ½ ripe avocado
- ¼ tsp turmeric
- 1 tbsp hemp seeds
- Lemon juice (optional)
- Salt and pepper to taste

1. Toast the bread.
2. Mash the avocado and mix in turmeric, salt, and pepper.
3. Spread the avocado mixture on the toast.
4. Sprinkle hemp seeds on top and add a drizzle of lemon juice if desired.

CHICKPEA FLOUR CREPES WITH SPICED VEGGIES

VG, GF, DF, SF, NF, V

PREP TIME: 10 mins   **COOK TIME:** 15 mins   **SERVINGS:** 2

CALORIES: 230 | CARBS: 32G | FAT: 5G | PROTEIN: 9G | FIBER: 6G

- ½ cup chickpea flour
- 1 cup water
- ½ tsp turmeric
- ¼ tsp salt
- ¼ tsp chili powder
- ½ cup mixed sautéed vegetables (onion, zucchini, bell peppers)
- 1 tbsp chopped fresh parsley

1. Whisk chickpea flour, water, turmeric, salt, and chili powder.
2. Cook as thin crepes on a greased skillet. Fill with sautéed veggies and parsley.

APPLE CINNAMON QUINOA PORRIDGE

VG, GF, DF, SF, V

PREP TIME: 5 mins   **COOK TIME:** 15 mins   **SERVINGS:** 2

CALORIES: 300 | CARBS: 50G | FAT: 8G | PROTEIN: 7G | FIBER: 5G

- ½ cup quinoa
- 1 cup almond milk
- 1 apple, diced
- 1 tbsp maple syrup
- ½ tsp cinnamon
- 1 tbsp raisins
- 1 tbsp crushed walnuts

1. Cook quinoa in almond milk until soft.
2. Stir in apples, raisins, maple syrup, and cinnamon. Simmer until apples are tender.
3. Garnish with walnuts before serving.

VEGAN PANCAKES WITH ORANGE ZEST AND CHOCOLATE CHIPS

VG, DF, SF, V

PREP TIME: 5 mins   **COOK TIME:** 15 mins

SERVINGS: 4 small pancakes

CALORIES: 160 | CARBS: 28G | FAT: 4G | PROTEIN: 3G | FIBER: 2G

- ½ cup whole-grain flour
- ½ cup almond milk
- 1 tbsp orange zest
- 1 tbsp maple syrup
- 1 tbsp dairy-free chocolate chips

1. Mix flour, milk, orange zest, and maple syrup. Stir in chocolate chips.
2. Cook pancakes on a greased skillet until golden.

HERB-INFUSED POACHED EGGS ON MUSHROOM TOAST

GF, SF, NF

PREP TIME: 5 mins   **COOK TIME:** 15 mins   **SERVINGS:** 2

CALORIES: 320 | CARBS: 36G | FAT: 11G | PROTEIN: 14G | FIBER: 4G

- 2 eggs
- 2 slices sourdough (GF bread)
- ½ cup sautéed mushrooms
- ¼ cup baby spinach
- 1 tsp fresh thyme
- 1 tsp white vinegar
- 1 tbsp grated Parmesan cheese

1. Poach eggs with thyme and vinegar in water.
2. Top toasted sourdough with mushrooms, spinach, Parmesan, and poached eggs.

PINEAPPLE SMOOTHIE WITH TURMERIC

VG, GF, SF, V

PREP TIME: 5 mins   **COOK TIME:** 0 min   **SERVINGS:** 1

CALORIES: 180 | PROTEIN: 3G | CARBS: 35G | FAT: 4G | FIBER: 6G

- 1 cup fresh or frozen pineapple chunks
- 1 ripe banana
- ½ tsp turmeric powder
- 1 tsp chia seeds
- 1 cup coconut water or almond milk
- 1 tbsp fresh ginger
- ½ tbsp honey or maple syrup

1. Blend all until smooth and creamy.
2. Pour into a glass and enjoy!

AVOCADO AND POMEGRANATE SALAD WRAP

VG, DF, SF, V

PREP TIME: 10 mins   **COOK TIME:** 5 mins   **SERVINGS:** 2

CALORIES: 280 | CARBS: 32G | FAT: 13G | PROTEIN: 6G | FIBER: 7G

- 1 avocado, sliced
- ¼ cup pomegranate seeds
- 2 whole-grain wraps
- 1 tbsp lemon juice
- 2 tbsp hummus
- ¼ cup shredded lettuce

1. Spread hummus on wraps, layer with avocado, pomegranate seeds, and lettuce.
2. Drizzle with lemon juice, roll tightly, and serve.

SWEET POTATO HASH WITH SPINACH

VG, GF, SF, DF, V

PREP TIME: 5 mins   **COOK TIME:** 15 mins   **SERVINGS:** 1

CALORIES: 230 | PROTEIN: 4G | CARBS: 35G | FAT: 10G | FIBER: 7G

- 1 small sweet potato, diced
- 1 cup fresh spinach
- 1 tbsp olive oil
- ½ red bell pepper, diced
- ¼ cup red onion, chopped
- 1 clove garlic, minced
- 1 tsp paprika
- ½ tsp cumin
- ¼ tsp turmeric
- Salt and pepper to taste
- Fresh herbs like parsley or cilantro for garnish

1. Heat olive oil in a pan and sauté diced sweet potatoes and red onion until tender (about 10 minutes).
2. Add red bell pepper and garlic, cooking for another 2-3 minutes until softened.
3. Stir in spinach, paprika, cumin, turmeric, salt, and pepper, cooking until the spinach wilts.
4. Garnish with fresh herbs like parsley or cilantro before serving.

SAVORY CHICKPEA PANCAKES WITH SPINACH

VG, GF, SF, V

PREP TIME: 15 mins   **COOK TIME:** 0 min   **SERVINGS:** 1

CALORIES: 220 | PROTEIN: 9G | CARBS: 25G | FAT: 10G | FIBER: 5G

- ½ cup chickpea flour
- ¼ cup water
- 1 cup fresh spinach, chopped
- 1 tbsp olive oil
- 1 garlic clove, minced
- ½ tsp cumin
- Pinch of chili flakes
- Salt and pepper, to taste

1. In a mixing bowl, combine chickpea flour, water, spinach, garlic, cumin, chili flakes, salt, and pepper. Stir to form a batter.
2. Heat olive oil in a non-stick pan over medium heat.
3. Pour in the batter to form small pancakes.
4. Cook each side for 3–4 minutes, or until golden brown and crispy on the edges.
5. Serve warm, topped with a sprinkle of fresh herbs or a squeeze of lemon juice for extra zest.

QUINOA BREAKFAST BOWL WITH ALMONDS AND POMEGRANATE

VG, GF, SF, V

PREP TIME: 15 mins   **COOK TIME:** 15 mins   **SERVINGS:** 1

CALORIES: 320 | PROTEIN: 9G | CARBS: 50G | FAT: 11G | FIBER: 7G

- ½ cup cooked quinoa (about ¼ cup uncooked quinoa)
- 1 tbsp ground pumpkin seeds
- ½ cup fresh blueberries
- 1 tsp honey or maple syrup
- 1 tsp vanilla extract
- 1 kiwi, sliced
- ½ tsp cinnamon
- 1 tbsp almond butter or peanut butter
- 1 tbsp chopped nuts (e.g., walnuts or almonds)
- 1 tbsp pomegranate seeds
- 1 tbsp sliced almonds
- Fresh mint leaves

1. Rinse the quinoa under cold water and cook it according to package (typically 1 part quinoa to 2 parts water). Bring to a boil, then cover and reduce the heat to a simmer for about 15 minutes. Once cooked, fluff with a fork and let it cool slightly.
2. In a bowl, combine the cooked quinoa, pumpkin seeds, and chopped nuts (walnuts or almonds). Add honey or maple syrup, then add the vanilla extract and cinnamon. Stir well to combine.
3. Top the quinoa mixture with fresh blueberries, pomegranate seeds, kiwi, and sliced almonds for crunch.
4. If desired, add a spoonful of almond butter (or peanut butter) and drizzle it over the top for added flavor.
5. Garnish with fresh mint leaves for a refreshing touch and extra flavor.

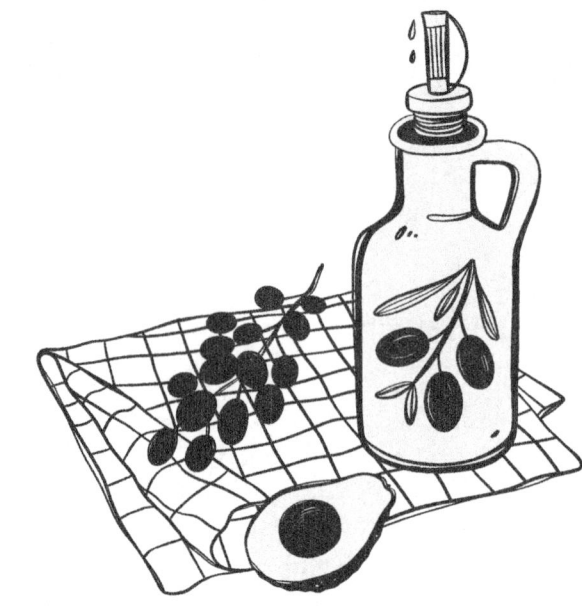

TOMATO AND BASIL BAKED EGGS WITH ARTICHOKES

GF, DF (OPTIONAL), SF, NF

PREP TIME: 10 mins   **COOK TIME:** 20 mins   **SERVINGS:** 2

CALORIES: 210 | CARBS: 7G | FAT: 15G | PROTEIN: 10G | FIBER: 2G

- 2 eggs
- 1/2 cup diced tomatoes
- 1 tbsp fresh basil
- 1 tbsp olive oil
- 1/4 cup chopped artichoke hearts

1. Heat tomatoes and artichokes in olive oil, transfer to a baking dish.
2. Crack eggs over the mixture and bake at 180°C for 10–15 minutes.

CURRIED TOFU SCRAMBLE

VG, GF, DF, SF, NF, V

PREP TIME: 10 mins   **COOK TIME:** 10 mins   **SERVINGS:** 2

CALORIES: 170 | CARBS: 10G | FAT: 8G | PROTEIN: 15G | FIBER: 3G

- 200 g tofu, crumbled
- 1/2 tsp curry powder
- 1/4 tsp turmeric
- 1/2 cup diced bell peppers
- 1/4 cup green peas
- 1 tbsp coconut milk

1. Sauté tofu with spices, bell peppers, and peas.
2. Stir in coconut milk and cook until creamy.

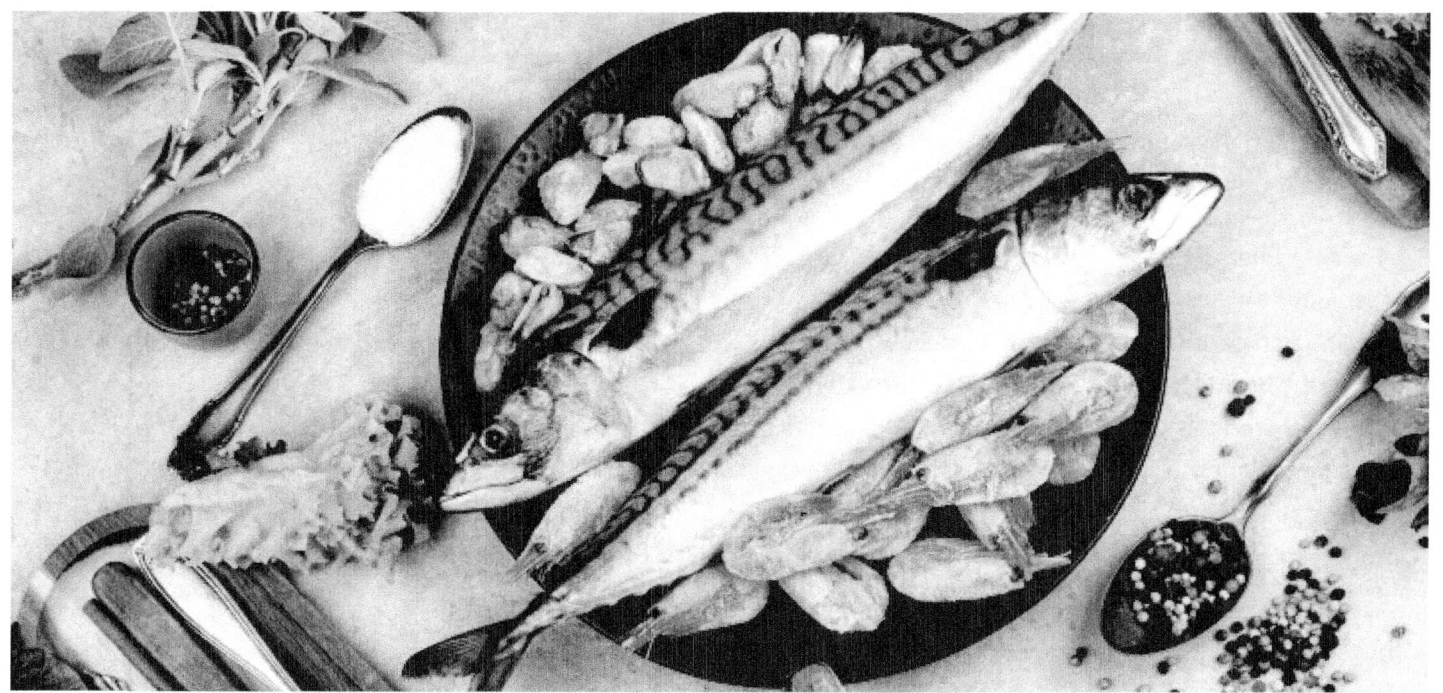

CHAPTER 8

FISH AND SEAFOOD

"From the sea, the power to soothe inflammation and restore your balance."

Fish and seafood are excellent sources of omega-3 fatty acids, which are powerful anti-inflammatory compounds.

These beneficial fats help reduce inflammation, decrease the risk of heart disease, and promote cognitive health.

Adding fish and seafood to an anti-inflammatory diet strengthens the immune system, supports heart health, and alleviates inflammation.

TIPS:

- **HEALTHY OPTIONS:** Opt for fatty fish like salmon, tuna, and mackerel, which are rich in omega-3s.

- **HERBS AND SPICES:** Use herbs and spices like turmeric, ginger, and garlic for added anti-inflammatory benefits.

- **STORAGE:** Fresh fish should be stored in the fridge and consumed within 1-2 days. Cooked fish can be refrigerated for up to 3 days in an airtight container.

BAKED GROUPER WITH ROASTED VEGETABLES

GF, DF

PREP TIME: 5 mins **COOK TIME:** 25 mins **SERVINGS:** 2

CALORIES: 360 | PROTEIN: 30G | CARBS: 16G | FAT: 18G | FIBER: 5G

- 2 Grouper fillets
- 1 tbsp olive oil
- 1 tsp smoked paprika
- 1 tsp garlic powder
- 1 tsp dried oregano
- 1 tbsp lemon juice
- 1 small sweet potato, cut into wedges
- 1 red bell pepper, diced
- 1 cup broccoli florets
- 1 carrot, sliced
- Salt and pepper, to taste
- Fresh parsley, chopped, for garnish

1. Preheat oven to 200°C (400°F).
2. Toss the sweet potato, bell pepper, broccoli, and carrot with half the olive oil, salt, and pepper. Spread on a baking tray lined with foil.
3. Place the grouper fillets on another sheet of foil. Rub with olive oil, smoked paprika, garlic powder, oregano, lemon juice, salt, and pepper. Seal the foil into a packet.
4. Bake vegetables and grouper together for 20-25 minutes or until the fish flakes easily with a fork and vegetables are tender.
5. Garnish with parsley and serve warm.

SEARED SCALLOPS WITH GARLIC SPINACH

GF, DF

PREP TIME: 10 mins **COOK TIME:** 10 mins **SERVINGS:** 2

CALORIES: 350 | PROTEIN: 30G | CARBS: 10G | FAT: 18G | FIBER: 4G

- 1 lb. (450 g) large sea scallops (about 12 scallops)
- 1 tbsp olive oil
- 1 tbsp ghee (or coconut oil for dairy-free)
- 3 garlic cloves, minced
- 6 cups fresh spinach
- Zest of 1 lemon
- 2 tbsp white wine or vegetable broth
- ¼ cup cherry tomatoes, halved
- Fresh basil or parsley, chopped
- Salt and pepper to taste
- Optional: Red pepper flakes for heat

1. Pat scallops dry, season with salt and pepper. Heat olive oil and ghee in a skillet, then sear scallops for 2-3 minutes per side until golden. Remove and set aside.
2. In the same skillet, cook garlic for 30 seconds, then deglaze with white wine or broth.
3. Add cherry tomatoes and sauté for 1 minute, then stir in spinach until wilted. Mix in lemon juice, zest, and red pepper flakes. Season with salt and pepper.
4. Serve spinach topped with seared scallops. Garnish with fresh herbs and drizzle with pan juices.

THAI COCONUT CURRY FISH

GF, DF, SF, NF

PREP TIME: 10 mins **COOK TIME:** 20 mins **SERVINGS:** 2

CALORIES: 340 | CARBS: 7G | FAT: 21G | PROTEIN: 31G | FIBER: 2G

- 2 white fish fillets (such as snapper or tilapia)
- 1 tbsp red curry paste
- 1 cup coconut milk
- 2 medium eggplant
- ¼ cup sliced onion
- 1 tbsp fish sauce
- ½ tsp grated lime zest
- 1 tsp fresh lime juice
- 1 tbsp chopped cilantro

1. Heat curry paste in a pan until fragrant, then stir in coconut milk.
2. Add fish fillets, eggplant, and onion. Simmer for 10–12 minutes or until fish is cooked through.
3. Stir in fish sauce, lime zest, and lime juice. Garnish with cilantro and serve.

SPICY GRILLED MACKEREL

GF, SF, DF, NF

PREP TIME: 5 mins **COOK TIME:** 20 mins **SERVINGS:** 2

CALORIES: 320 | PROTEIN: 25G | CARBS: 1G | FAT: 20G | FIBER: 0G

- 2 mackerel fillets
- 1 tbsp olive oil
- 1 tsp smoked paprika
- 1 tsp cayenne pepper
- 1 garlic clove, minced
- 1 tbsp lemon juice
- 1 tsp dried oregano
- Fresh parsley, chopped
- Salt and pepper to taste

1. Rub mackerel fillets with olive oil, garlic, smoked paprika, cayenne, lemon juice, lemon zest, oregano, salt, and pepper.
2. Grill fillets on medium heat for 6-8 minutes per side, until cooked through.
3. Garnish with fresh parsley before serving.

PESTO BAKED SALMON

GF, SF, DF, NF

PREP TIME: 5 mins **COOK TIME:** 20 mins **SERVINGS:** 2

CALORIES: 350 | PROTEIN: 30G | CARBS: 3G | FAT: 22G | FIBER: 1G

- 2 salmon fillets
- 2 tbsp pesto (homemade or store-bought)
- 1 tbsp olive oil
- 1 lemon, sliced
- ¼ cup cherry tomatoes, halved
- 1 tbsp capers
- Salt and pepper to taste

1. Preheat oven to 400°F (200°C).
2. Place salmon fillets in a baking dish. Top with pesto, drizzle with olive oil, and add lemon slices and cherry tomatoes around the salmon. Scatter capers on top.
3. Bake for 15-18 minutes until salmon flakes easily.

BLACKENED FISH TACOS

DF, SF, NF

PREP TIME: 10 mins **COOK TIME:** 15 mins **SERVINGS:** 2

CALORIES: 310 | CARBS: 28G | FAT: 8G | PROTEIN: 30G | FIBER: 4G

- 300 g white fish (tilapia or mahi-mahi)
- 1 tsp smoked paprika
- 1 tsp chili powder
- ½ tsp garlic powder
- ½ tsp cumin
- 4 small corn tortillas
- ½ cup shredded cabbage
- 2 tbsp diced red onion
- 1 tbsp lime juice
- 2 tbsp vegan mayo

1. Rub fish with spices and pan-sear for 3–4 minutes per side.
2. Fill tortillas with fish, cabbage, onion, and a drizzle of lime mayo.

GARLIC PARMESAN BAKED TILAPIA

GF, SF, NF

PREP TIME: 10 mins **COOK TIME:** 20 mins **SERVINGS:** 2

CALORIES: 290 | CARBS: 2G | FAT: 14G | PROTEIN: 38G | FIBER: 0G

- 2 tilapia fillets (150 g each)
- ¼ cup grated Parmesan cheese
- ½ tsp garlic powder
- ¼ tsp black pepper
- 1 tbsp olive oil
- 1 tbsp chopped parsley

1. Mix Parmesan, garlic powder, and black pepper. Coat tilapia fillets with olive oil and press the cheese mixture onto them.
2. Bake at 190°C (375°F) for 18–20 minutes until golden. Garnish with parsley.

SESAME GINGER GRILLED TROUT

GF, DF

PREP TIME: 10 mins **COOK TIME:** 15 mins **SERVINGS:** 2

CALORIES: 290 | CARBS: 3G | FAT: 15G | PROTEIN: 34G | FIBER: 0G

- 2 trout fillets (150 g each)
- 2 tbsp soy sauce (or tamari for GF)
- 1 tsp sesame oil
- ½ tsp grated ginger
- 1 tsp honey (or maple syrup for DF)
- 1 tsp sesame seeds

1. Marinate trout fillets in soy sauce, sesame oil, ginger, and honey for 10 minutes.
2. Grill fillets skin-side down for 6–7 minutes until cooked through.
3. Sprinkle with sesame seeds and serve warm.

SARDINES IN TOMATO SAUCE

GF, DF

PREP TIME: 5 mins **COOK TIME:** 20 mins **SERVINGS:** 2

CALORIES: 320 | PROTEIN: 24G | CARBS: 10G | FAT: 16G | FIBER: 3G

- 2 fresh sardines, cleaned
- 1 tbsp olive oil
- 2 shallots, thinly sliced
- 2 garlic cloves, minced
- 2 red chilies, sliced
- 200g canned diced tomatoes
- 1 tbsp tomato paste
- 1 tsp sugar (optional)
- 1 tbsp fish sauce
- 1 lemongrass stalk, thinly sliced
- 1 tbsp fresh kaffir lime leaves, shredded
- Fresh mint leaves, for garnish

1. Heat olive oil in a pan over medium heat. Sauté shallots, garlic, and chilies until fragrant.
2. Add diced tomatoes, tomato paste, sugar (if using), fish sauce, and lemongrass. Simmer for 5-7 minutes.
3. Add sardines to the pan, spooning the sauce over them. Cover and simmer for 10-12 minutes until the fish is cooked through.
4. Stir in kaffir lime leaves and adjust seasoning with salt and pepper if needed.
5. Garnish with fresh mint leaves and serve warm.

SPICY CRAB MEAT STUFFED PEPPERS

GF, DF, SF, NF

PREP TIME: 10 mins **COOK TIME:** 20 mins **SERVINGS:** 2

CALORIES: 230 | CARBS: 9G | FAT: 11G | PROTEIN: 23G | FIBER: 3G

- 2 bell peppers, halved and deseeded
- 1 cup crab meat
- ¼ cup diced celery
- ¼ cup chopped onion
- 1 tbsp mayonnaise (or vegan mayo for DF)
- ½ tsp smoked paprika
- ½ tsp chili flakes
- 1 tbsp breadcrumbs (GF option available)

1. Mix crab meat, celery, onion, mayonnaise, paprika, and chili flakes.
2. Stuff the mixture into the halved bell peppers and sprinkle with breadcrumbs.
3. Bake at 190°C (375°F) for 15–20 minutes until the peppers are tender.

SPICY CRISPY CALAMARI WITH LIME DIP

DF, SF, NF

PREP TIME: 10 mins **COOK TIME:** 20 mins **SERVINGS:** 2

CALORIES: 260 | CARBS: 22G | FAT: 10G | PROTEIN: 17G | FIBER: 1G

- 200 g calamari rings
- ¼ cup rice flour
- ¼ cup cornstarch
- ½ tsp cayenne pepper
- ½ tsp garlic powder
- Oil for frying
- Lime wedges for serving

1. Coat calamari in a mix of rice flour, cornstarch, cayenne, and garlic powder.
2. Fry in hot oil until golden and crispy. Serve with lime wedges.

BAKED HERB CRUSTED HALIBUT

GF, DF, SF

PREP TIME: 10 mins **COOK TIME:** 15 mins **SERVINGS:** 2

CALORIES: 290 | CARBS: 3G | FAT: 12G | PROTEIN: 40G | FIBER: 1G

- 2 halibut fillets (150 g each)
- 2 tbsp almond flour
- 1 tbsp chopped parsley
- ½ tsp garlic powder
- ½ tsp lemon zest
- 1 tbsp olive oil

1. Mix almond flour, parsley, garlic powder, and lemon zest. Coat halibut with olive oil and press herb mixture onto fillets.
2. Bake at 200°C (400°F) for 12–15 minutes.

CHILI GARLIC MUSSELS IN TOMATO BROTH

GF, DF, NF

PREP TIME: 5 mins **COOK TIME:** 20 mins **SERVINGS:** 2

- 500 g mussels, cleaned
- 2 tbsp olive oil
- 3 garlic cloves, minced
- ¼ tsp red chili flakes
- ½ cup diced tomatoes
- ¼ cup white wine (or vegetable broth for DF)
- 2 tbsp fresh parsley

1. Heat olive oil, sauté garlic and chili flakes, then add tomatoes.
2. Stir in white wine, bring to a boil, and add mussels. Cover.

SEA BASS WITH GREEK SALAD

GF, DF

PREP TIME: 10 mins **COOK TIME:** 20 mins **SERVINGS:** 2

CALORIES: 320 | PROTEIN: 35G | CARBS: 12G | FAT: 15G | FIBER: 4G

- 2 sea bass fillets (200g each)
- 1 tbsp olive oil
- 1 tsp dried oregano
- 1 tsp fresh garlic, minced
- ½ tsp paprika
- Salt and pepper to taste
- 1 cucumber, diced
- 1 large tomato, diced
- ½ red onion, sliced
- 10 black olives, halved
- 50g feta cheese (optional), cubed
- 1 tbsp olive oil
- 1 tsp red wine vinegar
- 1 tsp fresh dill or parsley, chopped

1. Preheat your oven to 200°C (400°F).
2. Brush the sea bass fillets with olive oil. Sprinkle with oregano, garlic, paprika, salt, and pepper.
3. Place the fillets on a baking tray lined with parchment paper. Bake for 15-20 minutes or until the fish flakes easily with a fork.
4. While the fish is baking, prepare the Greek salad by mixing cucumber, tomato, red onion, olives, and feta (if using).
5. Drizzle olive oil and red wine vinegar over the salad. Toss with fresh dill or parsley.
6. Serve the baked sea bass alongside the fresh Greek salad.

LEMONGRASS FISH SKEWERS

GF, DF, SF, NF

PREP TIME: 10 mins **COOK TIME:** 15 mins **SERVINGS:** 2

CALORIES: 230 | CARBS: 1G | FAT: 6G | PROTEIN: 38G | FIBER: 0G

- 300 g white fish (cod or tilapia), cubed
- 2 lemongrass stalks, trimmed
- 1 tbsp lime juice
- 1 tsp grated ginger
- ½ tsp chili flakes
- ¼ tsp freshly ground black pepper

1. Thread fish cubes onto lemongrass stalks. Marinate with lime, ginger, black pepper and chili flakes for 10 minutes.
2. Grill skewers for 3–4 minutes per side.

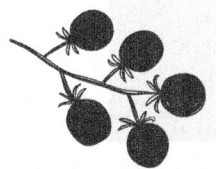

TUNA SALAD LETTUCE WRAPS

GF, SF, DF, NF

PREP TIME: 10 mins **COOK TIME:** 0 min **SERVINGS:** 2

CALORIES: 269 | PROTEIN: 34G | CARBS: 8G | FAT: 11G | FIBER: 5G

- 1 can tuna (in water), drained
- 1 tbsp olive oil mayo
- 1 tsp Dijon mustard
- 1 celery stalk, chopped
- 1 tbsp fresh parsley, chopped
- Romaine lettuce leaves (large)
- ¼ cup diced red bell pepper
- ¼ cup diced carrots
- 1 tbsp capers
- 1 tsp lemon juice
- Salt and pepper

1. In a bowl, mix tuna, mayo, mustard, celery, parsley, red bell pepper, carrots, capers, lemon juice, salt, and pepper.
2. Spoon the tuna salad onto romaine lettuce leaves and roll them up.

GRILLED SALMON WITH AVOCADO SALSA

GF, SF, DF, NF

PREP TIME: 10 mins **COOK TIME:** 10 mins **SERVINGS:** 2

CALORIES: 350 | PROTEIN: 30G | CARBS: 24G | FAT: 10G | FIBER: 7G

- 2 salmon fillets
- 1 ripe avocado, diced
- 1 small tomato, diced
- ¼ red onion, diced
- 1 tbsp lime juice
- 1 tbsp olive oil
- ¼ cup fresh cilantro, chopped
- ½ jalapeño, finely chopped
- 1 clove garlic, minced
- Zest of 1 lime
- Salt and pepper to taste

1. Preheat grill to medium heat.
2. Season salmon with olive oil, salt, and pepper. Grill for 4-5 minutes per side.
3. In a bowl, mix avocado, tomato, red onion, cilantro, jalapeño, garlic, lime juice, lime zest, and a pinch of salt to prepare the salsa.
4. Serve salmon topped with the flavorful avocado salsa.

LEMON GARLIC BAKED THYME COD

GF, SF, DF

PREP TIME: 5 mins **COOK TIME:** 20 mins **SERVINGS:** 2

CALORIES: 220 | PROTEIN: 28G | CARBS: 2G | FAT: 10G | FIBER: 0G

- 2 cod fillets
- 2 tbsp olive oil
- 2 garlic cloves, minced
- Juice of 1 lemon
- 1 tbsp fresh parsley, chopped
- ¼ tsp paprika
- ¼ tsp dried thyme
- ½ tsp Dijon mustard
- Salt and pepper

1. Preheat oven to 400°F (200°C).
2. In a small bowl, mix olive oil, garlic, lemon juice, Dijon mustard, paprika, thyme, and lemon zest.
3. Place cod fillets in a baking dish and pour the seasoning mixture over the fish. Season with salt and pepper.
4. Bake for 15-18 minutes until the fish flakes easily with a fork.
5. Garnish with fresh parsley before serving.

SHRIMP STIR-FRY WITH VEGETABLES

GF, SF, DF, NF

PREP TIME: 10 mins **COOK TIME:** 10 mins **SERVINGS:** 2

CALORIES: 230 | PROTEIN: 28G | CARBS: 10G | FAT: 9G | FIBER: 3G

- 200g shrimp, peeled and deveined
- 1 tsp turmeric powder
- 1 tsp fresh grated ginger
- 1 garlic clove, minced
- 1 tbsp olive oil
- 1 bell pepper, sliced
- 1 zucchini, sliced
- 1 cup broccoli florets
- Salt and pepper to taste

1. Heat olive oil in a pan over medium-high heat.
2. Add the bell pepper, zucchini, and broccoli to the pan. Sauté for 4-5 minutes until slightly tender.
3. Move the vegetables to the side of the pan and add the shrimp, turmeric, ginger, and garlic to the center.
4. Sauté the shrimp for 3-4 minutes until pink and cooked through, mixing everything together for the last minute to combine flavors.
5. Season with salt and pepper.
6. Squeeze a little lime juice before serving.

CREOLE FISH STEW

GF, DF, SF, NF

PREP TIME: 10 mins **COOK TIME:** 20 mins **SERVINGS:** 2

CALORIES: 250 | CARBS: 8G | FAT: 6G | PROTEIN: 40G | FIBER: 2G

- 300 g white fish fillets, cubed
- ½ cup diced bell peppers
- ¼ cup diced celery
- ¼ cup diced onion
- ¼ cup diced tomatoes
- 1 tsp Creole seasoning blend
- ½ cup vegetable broth
- Creole Seasoning Blend
- 1 tsp paprika
- ½ tsp onion powder
- ½ tsp garlic powder
- ½ tsp thyme
- ¼ tsp cayenne pepper
- ¼ tsp oregano
- ¼ tsp black pepper
- ¼ tsp salt

1. Sauté onion, celery, and bell peppers. Add Creole seasoning and tomatoes.
2. Pour in broth and simmer fish for 8–10 minutes until tender.

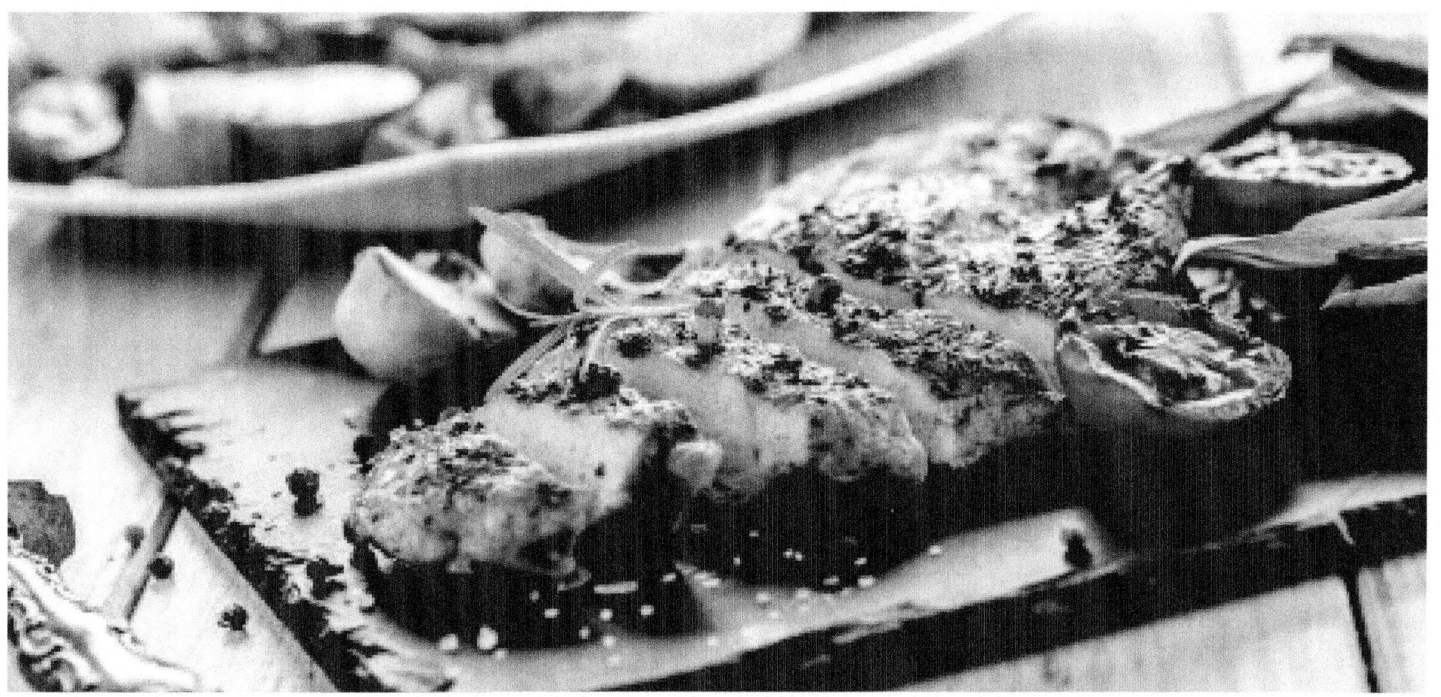

CHAPTER 9

MEAT AND POULTRY

"Lean into invigorating health with every bite of clean, nutrient-rich protein."

Meat and poultry recipes focus on lean cuts like skinless chicken, turkey, and grass-fed beef, which are rich in protein and healthy fats.

These dishes often include herbs and spices like turmeric, garlic, and rosemary to boost their anti-inflammatory effects.

Grilling, baking, or slow-cooking are preferred methods to retain nutrients.

TIPS:

- **MEAT:** Choose organic, hormone-free meat and poultry for cleaner options.

- **HERBS AND SPICES:** Add herbs, spices, and healthy oils like olive oil for added benefits.

- **STORAGE:** Store cooked meat in airtight containers in the fridge for up to 3-4 days. Freeze any leftovers in portions to maintain freshness for up to 2-3 months.

GOLDEN GRILLED CHICKEN

GF, DF, NF

PREP TIME: 10 mins **COOK TIME:** 20 mins **SERVINGS:** 2

CALORIES: 280 | PROTEIN: 35G | CARBS: 3G | FAT: 12G | FIBER: 2G

- 2 chicken breasts
- 1 tsp turmeric
- 1 tsp garlic powder
- 2 tbsp olive oil
- 1 tsp lemon juice
- 1 tsp honey
- ½ tsp paprika
- Fresh parsley, chopped (for garnish)
- Salt and pepper to taste

1. Mix turmeric, garlic powder, olive oil, lemon juice, honey, paprika, salt, and pepper into a paste.
2. Coat the chicken breasts with the paste and grill on medium heat for 6–7 minutes per side until cooked through.
3. Garnish with fresh parsley before serving.

CILANTRO-LIME GRILLED PORK CHOPS

GF, SF, NF, DF

PREP TIME: 5 mins **COOK TIME:** 10 mins **SERVINGS:** 4

CALORIES: 320 | PROTEIN: 35G | CARBS: 12G | FAT: 12G | FIBER: 1G

- 4 pork chops
- ¼ cup lime juice
- Zest of 1 lime
- 2 tbsp fresh cilantro, chopped
- 1 tbsp olive oil
- 2 garlic cloves, minced
- 1 tsp cumin
- ¼ tsp chili powder
- Salt and pepper to taste
- Fresh cilantro leaves

1. In a bowl, marinate the pork chops with lime juice, lime zest, cilantro, olive oil, garlic, cumin, chili powder, salt, and pepper for 5 minutes.
2. Grill the pork chops for 5–6 minutes on each side until fully cooked and nicely charred.
3. Serve with a green salad and garnish with fresh cilantro for added freshness.

HERB-CITRUS TURKEY SKEWERS

GF, DF, SF, NF

PREP TIME: 10 mins **COOK TIME:** 10 mins **SERVINGS:** 4

CALORIES: 270 | PROTEIN: 30G | CARBS: 5G | FAT: 10G | FIBER: 1G

- 1 lb. turkey breast, cubed
- 2 tbsp lemon juice
- Zest of 1 lemon
- 1 tsp Dijon mustard
- 1 tbsp olive oil
- 1 tbsp honey or maple syrup
- 1 tsp ground coriander
- 1 tbsp fresh rosemary, chopped
- 2 garlic cloves, minced
- Salt and pepper to taste
- Fresh parsley, chopped (for garnish)

1. Combine lemon juice, zest, Dijon mustard, olive oil, honey, ground coriander, rosemary, garlic, salt, and pepper in a bowl. Mix well.
2. Add turkey cubes to the marinade and let sit for 10 minutes.
3. Thread the turkey onto skewers and grill over medium heat for 3–4 minutes on each side, or until fully cooked.
4. Serve with a side of roasted vegetables or couscous. Garnish with fresh parsley before serving.

HERB CRUSTED CHICKEN CUTLETS

GF, SF

PREP TIME: 10 mins **COOK TIME:** 15 mins **SERVINGS:** 2

CALORIES: 300 | CARBS: 4G | FAT: 14G | PROTEIN: 38G | FIBER: 1G

- 2 chicken cutlets
- ¼ cup almond flour
- ¼ cup grated Parmesan
- 1 tsp Italian herb seasoning blend
- ½ tsp garlic powder
- Italian Herb Seasoning Blend
- 1 tsp dried oregano
- 1 tsp dried basil
- ½ tsp dried thyme
- ½ tsp garlic powder
- ¼ tsp onion powder
- ¼ tsp red pepper flakes

1. In a shallow bowl, mix almond flour, Parmesan, Italian seasoning, and garlic powder.
2. Coat each chicken cutlet in the mixture, pressing gently to ensure it sticks.
3. Heat a non-stick skillet over medium heat and pan-fry the chicken for 5–7 minutes per side, or until golden brown and cooked through.

HONEY MUSTARD CHICKEN DRUMSTICKS

GF, DF, SF, NF

PREP TIME: 10 mins **COOK TIME:** 20 mins **SERVINGS:** 2
CALORIES: 300 | CARBS: 8G | FAT: 14G | PROTEIN: 36G | FIBER: 0G

- 4 chicken drumsticks
- 1 tbsp honey
- 1 tbsp Dijon mustard
- 1 tbsp olive oil
- 1 garlic clove, minced

1. Coat drumsticks with honey, mustard, olive oil, and garlic.
2. Bake at 200°C (400°F) for 20 minutes, turning halfway through.

SWEET AND SOUR TURKEY MEATBALLS

GF, DF

PREP TIME: 10 mins **COOK TIME:** 20 mins **SERVINGS:** 2
CALORIES: 280 | CARBS: 10G | FAT: 10G | PROTEIN: 34G | FIBER: 1G

- 300 g ground turkey
- ¼ cup almond flour
- 1 egg
- 1 tbsp soy sauce (or tamari for GF)
- ¼ cup pineapple juice
- ¼ cup ketchup
- 1 tbsp vinegar

1. Form turkey into small meatballs. Sear in a skillet until browned.
2. Mix soy sauce, pineapple juice, ketchup, and vinegar, then pour over meatballs. Simmer for 10 minutes.

GROUND BEEF STIR-FRY

GF, DF, NF

PREP TIME: 10 mins **COOK TIME:** 15 mins **SERVINGS:** 2
CALORIES: 280 | CARBS: 6G | FAT: 18G | PROTEIN: 24G | FIBER: 1G

- 300 g ground beef
- ½ cup diced bell peppers
- ¼ cup sliced onions
- 1 tbsp soy sauce (or tamari for GF)
- ¼ tsp chili flakes

1. Brown ground beef in a skillet. Add onions, peppers, soy sauce, and chili flakes.
2. Cook for 5 minutes until vegetables are tender.

HARISSA ROASTED LAMB MEATBALLS

GF, DF, SF

PREP TIME: 10 mins **COOK TIME:** 20 mins **SERVINGS:** 2
CALORIES: 350 | CARBS: 4G | FAT: 22G | PROTEIN: 30G | FIBER: 1G

- 300 g ground lamb
- 1 tbsp harissa paste
- ½ tsp ground cumin
- ½ tsp smoked paprika
- 1 garlic clove, minced
- 2 tbsp chopped parsley
- ¼ cup almond flour

1. Preheat oven to 200°C (400°F). Mix all in a bowl and form into small meatballs.
2. Arrange on a baking tray and roast for 18–20 minutes until browned and cooked through and serve.

PEPPERCORN CRUSTED STEAK WITH GARLIC BUTTER

GF, SF, NF

PREP TIME: 10 mins **COOK TIME:** 15 mins **SERVINGS:** 2
CALORIES: 340 | CARBS: 1G | FAT: 24G | PROTEIN: 30G | FIBER: 0G

- 2 beef steaks (150 g each)
- 1 tbsp crushed black peppercorns
- 1 tsp salt
- 2 tbsp butter
- 2 garlic cloves, minced
- 1 tsp chopped thyme

1. Press crushed peppercorns onto both sides of the steak. Season with salt.
2. Heat a skillet and sear steaks for 3–4 minutes per side to desired doneness.
3. Melt butter in the skillet with garlic and thyme. Spoon over steaks before serving.

SPICED MOROCCAN GROUND LAMB

GF, DF, SF, NF

PREP TIME: 10 mins **COOK TIME:** 15 mins **SERVINGS:** 2
CALORIES: 320 | CARBS: 2G | FAT: 22G | PROTEIN: 28G | FIBER: 0G

- 300 g ground lamb
- ½ tsp ground cinnamon
- ½ tsp ground cumin
- ¼ tsp smoked paprika
- 1 tbsp olive oil
- 2 tbsp chopped mint

1. Heat oil in a skillet and cook lamb with cinnamon, cumin, and paprika.
2. Garnish with chopped mint before serving.

THAI COCONUT CURRY CHICKEN

GF, DF, NF

PREP TIME: 5 mins **COOK TIME:** 25 mins **SERVINGS:** 2

CALORIES: 380 | PROTEIN: 32G | CARBS: 18G | FAT: 20G | FIBER: 3G

- 2 chicken breasts
- 1 tbsp olive oil
- 1 tbsp red curry paste
- ½ can (200ml) coconut milk (canned, full-fat)
- 1 tbsp lime juice
- 1 tsp garlic powder
- 1 tsp ground turmeric
- 1 tsp ground ginger
- Salt and pepper to taste
- ½ cup mushrooms, sliced
- 1 small red bell pepper, sliced
- ½ cup snap peas
- ½ cup baby spinach
- Fresh cilantro, chopped, for garnish

1. Heat olive oil in a large skillet over medium heat. Season the chicken breasts with salt, pepper, garlic powder, turmeric, and ground ginger.
2. Once the skillet is hot, add the chicken breasts and sear them for about 3–4 minutes per side, until browned.
3. Add the red curry paste and coconut milk to the pan, stirring to combine. Bring the sauce to a simmer, reduce the heat, and cook the chicken for another 10–12 minutes, or until the chicken is cooked through.
4. Add the bell pepper, snap peas, mushrooms, and spinach to the skillet during the last 5 minutes of cooking, letting the vegetables soften.
5. Stir in lime juice, adjust seasoning if needed. Garnish with fresh cilantro and serve warm.

CUMIN-SPICED BEEF TACOS

GF, DF, NF

PREP TIME: 10 mins **COOK TIME:** 20 mins **SERVINGS:** 4

CALORIES: 350 | PROTEIN: 25G | CARBS: 22G | FAT: 18G | FIBER: 6G

- 1 lb. lean ground beef
- 1 tbsp cumin powder
- ½ tsp smoked paprika
- ½ tsp chili powder
- 2 garlic cloves, minced
- 8 small corn tortillas
- 1 avocado, sliced
- 1 cup shredded lettuce
- 1 tomato, diced
- ¼ cup red onion, finely chopped
- Fresh cilantro, chopped
- Salt and pepper to taste

1. Heat a pan over medium heat, add the ground beef, and cook for 7–8 minutes until browned.
2. Stir in cumin, smoked paprika, chili powder, garlic, salt, and pepper. Cook for another 2 minutes.
3. Serve the beef mixture in corn tortillas with avocado, lettuce, tomato, red onion, and a sprinkle of cilantro.

HONEY GARLIC CHICKEN THIGHS

GF, DF, NF

PREP TIME: 10 mins **COOK TIME:** 20 mins **SERVINGS:** 2

CALORIES: 320 | CARBS: 14G | FAT: 18G | PROTEIN: 28G | FIBER: 0G

- 4 chicken thighs (bone-in or boneless)
- 2 tbsp honey
- 2 tbsp soy sauce (or tamari for GF)
- 1 tbsp rice vinegar
- 2 garlic cloves, minced
- ½ tsp grated ginger
- ¼ tsp chili flakes
- 1 tbsp olive oil

1. Heat oil in a skillet and sear chicken thighs for 4–5 minutes per side until golden brown.
2. Mix honey, soy sauce, rice vinegar, garlic, ginger, and chili flakes in a bowl.
3. Pour the sauce into the skillet, reduce heat, and simmer for 10 minutes until the chicken is cooked and the sauce thickens.

LEMON-HERB LAMB CHOPS

GF, SF, NF, DF

PREP TIME: 5 mins **COOK TIME:** 10 mins **SERVINGS:** 4

CALORIES: 360 | PROTEIN: 30G | CARBS: 5G | FAT: 20G | FIBER: 1G

- 4 lamb chops
- 2 tbsp lemon juice
- Zest of 1 lemon
- 1 tbsp fresh rosemary, chopped
- 1 tbsp olive oil
- 2 garlic cloves, minced
- 1 tsp Dijon mustard
- ½ tsp smoked paprika
- ½ tsp dried thyme
- Salt and pepper to taste
- Fresh parsley, chopped

1. In a bowl, mix lemon juice, lemon zest, rosemary, garlic, Dijon mustard, smoked paprika, thyme, olive oil, salt, and pepper to create the marinade. Marinate the lamb chops in the mixture for at least 5 minutes (or overnight for maximum flavor).
2. Grill the lamb chops for 5–6 minutes on each side until they reach your desired level of doneness.
3. Serve with a side of quinoa or roasted vegetables, and garnish with fresh parsley.

BALSAMIC GLAZED CHICKEN BREASTS

GF, SF, NF, DF

PREP TIME: 5 mins **COOK TIME:** 10 mins **SERVINGS:** 4

CALORIES: 330 | PROTEIN: 32G | CARBS: 3G | FAT: 18G | FIBER: 0G

- 4 chicken breasts
- ¼ cup balsamic vinegar
- 2 tbsp olive oil
- 1 tbsp honey
- 2 cloves garlic, minced
- 1 tsp dried rosemary or thyme
- ¼ tsp red pepper flakes
- Salt and pepper to taste
- Fresh basil or parsley, chopped (for garnish)

1. Heat olive oil in a pan over medium heat. Season the chicken breasts with salt, pepper, and dried rosemary or thyme. Cook the chicken for 6–7 minutes on each side until golden and cooked through.
2. Add minced garlic, balsamic vinegar, and honey to the pan. Simmer for 2–3 minutes until the sauce thickens and coats the chicken.
3. Serve the balsamic glazed chicken with a side of steamed vegetables and garnish with fresh basil or parsley.

PAPRIKA-RUBBED STEAK

GF, SF, NF, DF

PREP TIME: 5 mins **COOK TIME:** 10 mins **SERVINGS:** 4

CALORIES: 400 | PROTEIN: 35G | CARBS: 3G | FAT: 25G | FIBER: 1G

- 4 beef steaks
- 1 tbsp paprika
- 1 tbsp olive oil
- 1 tsp garlic powder
- 1 tsp onion powder
- 1 tsp dried oregano
- Salt and pepper to taste
- Fresh parsley, chopped (for garnish)

1. Rub the steaks with olive oil, paprika, garlic powder, onion powder, oregano, salt, and pepper.
2. Grill the steaks for 4–5 minutes on each side until desired doneness.
3. Serve with roasted vegetables and garnish with fresh parsley.

GARLIC ROSEMARY PORK TENDERLOIN

GF, DF, SF, NF

PREP TIME: 10 mins **COOK TIME:** 20 mins **SERVINGS:** 2

CALORIES: 240 | CARBS: 2G | FAT: 8G | PROTEIN: 36G | FIBER: 0G

- 1 pork tenderloin (300 g)
- 1 tbsp olive oil
- 2 garlic cloves, minced
- 1 tsp chopped rosemary
- ½ tsp smoked paprika
- ¼ tsp ground pepper

1. Rub tenderloin with olive oil, garlic, rosemary, paprika, and pepper.
2. Sear in a hot skillet for 2–3 minutes per side, then bake at 200°C (400°F) for 12–15 minutes.

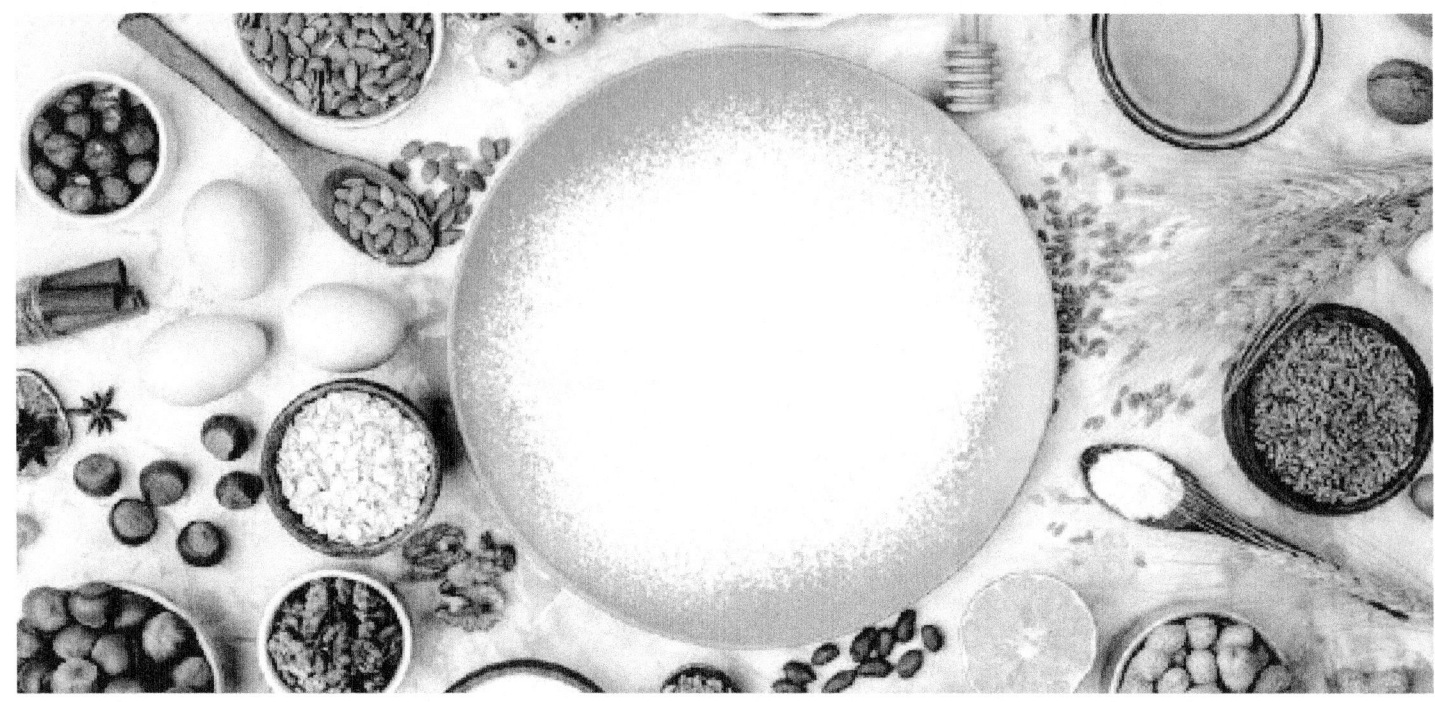

CHAPTER 10

EGGS AND GRAINS

"Wholesome grains, hearty beginnings - every meal is an intentional step to embrace the strength within you."

Whole grains like quinoa, oats, and brown rice are rich in fiber and phytonutrients, which help reduce inflammation and balance blood sugar levels.

Eggs, an excellent source of choline, support brain health while also contributing to a reduction in inflammation.

Eggs may not sit well with everyone, especially if they have sensitivities that can impact gut health. It's always a good idea to check for any trigger foods that could cause discomfort.

TIPS:

- **WHOLE GRAINS:** Quinoa, millet, or oats to provide sustained energy and reduce inflammation.
- **PAIRING:** Accompany grains with vegetables and healthy fats like olive oil or avocado for a balanced meal.
- **STORAGE:** Store cooked grains and egg dishes in airtight containers in the fridge for up to 3 days. Reheat eggs and grains gently on the stovetop or microwave to preserve texture and flavor.

QUINOA BREAKFAST BOWL WITH POACHED EGGS AND AVOCADO

GF, DF, SF

PREP TIME: 5 mins **COOK TIME:** 10 mins **SERVINGS:** 4

CALORIES: 400 KCAL | PROTEIN: 20G | CARBS: 30G | FAT: 28G | FIBER: 8G

- 1 cup cooked quinoa
- 2 eggs (poached)
- 1 avocado, sliced
- ½ cup spinach
- 1 tbsp olive oil
- 1 tbsp lemon juice
- ¼ tsp red pepper flakes
- Salt and pepper to taste
- Fresh herbs (like cilantro or parsley) for garnish

1. Cook quinoa according to package.
2. Poach eggs in simmering water for 3–4 minutes until the whites are set.
3. In a bowl, layer quinoa, spinach, avocado slices, and poached eggs.
4. Drizzle with olive oil and lemon juice, and season with salt, pepper, and red pepper flakes.
5. Garnish with fresh herbs for an extra flavor boost.

ZUCCHINI QUINOA FRITTATA

GF, DF, SF

PREP TIME: 10 mins **COOK TIME:** 15 mins **SERVINGS:** 2

CALORIES: 320 KCAL | PROTEIN: 22G | CARBS: 24G | FAT: 18G | FIBER: 4G

- 1 cup cooked quinoa
- 4 eggs, whisked
- ½ bell pepper, diced
- ¼ zucchini, diced
- ¼ cup cherry tomatoes, halved
- 1 tbsp olive oil
- ¼ tsp dried oregano or thyme
- Salt and pepper to taste
- Fresh parsley or basil, chopped (for garnish)

1. Preheat the oven to 375°F (190°C).
2. In a skillet, heat olive oil and sauté the bell pepper, zucchini, and cherry tomatoes until softened.
3. Add the cooked quinoa, whisked eggs, and dried oregano or thyme to the skillet, mixing well.
4. Transfer the mixture to the oven and bake for 15 minutes or until set and lightly golden.
5. Garnish with fresh parsley or basil before serving.

STUFFED EGG WRAP WITH MINCED PORK AND VEGETABLES

GF, DF

PREP TIME: 10 mins **COOK TIME:** 15 mins **SERVINGS:** 2

CALORIES: 450 KCAL | PROTEIN: 35G | CARBS: 20G | FAT: 25G | FIBER: 5G

- 4 large eggs, beaten
- 200g (7 oz) minced pork
- ½ cup peas
- ½ cup diced carrots
- ¼ cup diced red bell pepper
- 1 tbsp soy sauce (use tamari for gluten-free)
- 1 tbsp olive oil
- 1 garlic clove, minced
- Salt and pepper to taste
- Fresh cilantro for garnish

1. Heat olive oil in a skillet over medium heat. Add garlic and sauté until fragrant.
2. Add minced pork to the skillet and cook until browned.
3. Stir in peas, carrots, and bell pepper. Cook for 3–4 minutes. Season with soy sauce, salt, and pepper. Set aside.
4. In a separate non-stick pan, pour half of the beaten eggs to form a thin, even layer. Cook for 2–3 minutes until set.
5. Place half of the pork and vegetable mixture in the center of the egg wrap. Fold the edges over to form a parcel. Repeat with the remaining eggs and filling. Garnish with fresh cilantro and serve warm.

SCRAMBLED EGG AND FARRO PILAF

DF, SF, NF

PREP TIME: 10 mins **COOK TIME:** 20 mins **SERVINGS:** 2

CALORIES: 330 | CARBS: 38G | FAT: 12G | PROTEIN: 14G | FIBER: 6G

- 1 cup cooked farro
- 2 large eggs
- ¼ cup diced carrots
- ¼ cup diced celery
- 1 tbsp olive oil
- ¼ tsp garlic powder
- ¼ tsp black pepper

1. Heat olive oil in a skillet and sauté carrots and celery for 5 minutes.
2. Add farro, garlic powder, and black pepper. Cook for 10 minutes.
3. Scramble eggs separately and mix into the farro. Serve warm.

RAMEN WITH SOFT-BOILED EGG AND TOFU

GF (USE GLUTEN FREE NOODLES), DF, NF

PREP TIME: 10 mins **COOK TIME:** 15 mins **SERVINGS:** 2

CALORIES: 400 KCAL | PROTEIN: 20G | CARBS: 50G | FAT: 10G | FIBER: 4G

- 2 packs of ramen noodles (MSG-free, gluten-free if preferred)
- 4 cups vegetable or chicken broth
- 1 tbsp sesame oil
- 2 cloves garlic, minced
- 1 tbsp soy sauce (or tamari for gluten-free)
- 1 tbsp chili paste (adjust to taste)
- ½ tsp ginger, grated
- ½ block of firm tofu, cubed
- 2 soft-boiled eggs, halved
- ¼ cup chopped green onions
- Optional: ½ tsp miso paste for added depth

4. Heat sesame oil in a pot over medium heat. Sauté garlic and ginger until fragrant.
5. Add chili paste, soy sauce, and broth. Bring to a simmer. Stir in miso paste (if using).
6. Add tofu cubes and simmer for 5 minutes.
7. Cook ramen noodles according to package and divide them into bowls.
8. Pour the hot broth with tofu over the noodles.
9. Top each bowl with soft-boiled egg halves, green onions, and extra chili paste if desired.

SWEET CORN EGG RISOTTO

DF, SF, NF

PREP TIME: 10 mins **COOK TIME:** 20 mins **SERVINGS:** 2

CALORIES: 340 | CARBS: 42G | FAT: 12G | PROTEIN: 13G | FIBER: 2G

- 1 cup cooked arborio rice
- 2 large eggs
- ¼ cup sweet corn kernels
- ¼ cup grated Parmesan cheese
- 1 tbsp butter

1. Heat butter in a skillet and stir in cooked rice and sweet corn.
2. Mix in Parmesan cheese and cook for 5 minutes.
3. Fry eggs and serve on top of the risotto.

EGG AND MILLET BOWL WITH SPINACH

GF, DF, SF

PREP TIME: 10 mins **COOK TIME:** 15 mins **SERVINGS:** 2

CALORIES: 330 KCAL | PROTEIN: 15G | CARBS: 35G | FAT: 14G | FIBER: 5G

- 1 cup cooked millet
- 2 eggs (boiled or fried)
- ½ cup spinach, sautéed
- 1 tbsp olive oil
- ¼ avocado, sliced
- 1 tsp lemon juice
- Salt and pepper to taste
- Fresh herbs like parsley or cilantro

1. Cook millet according to the package until fluffy.
2. In a skillet, sauté spinach in olive oil until wilted and cook the eggs to your liking (boiled or fried).
3. In a bowl, layer the millet, spinach, and eggs. Add avocado slices and a drizzle of lemon juice for extra flavor.
4. Garnish with fresh herbs and season with salt and pepper to taste.

CREAMY BACON & EGG SPAGHETTI

SF, NF

PREP TIME: 10 mins **COOK TIME:** 20 mins **SERVINGS:** 2

CALORIES: 600 KCAL | PROTEIN: 25G | CARBS: 45G | FAT: 25G | FIBER: 3G

- 200g spaghetti (or gluten-free option)
- 4 strips of bacon, cooked and chopped
- 2 eggs (fried sunny-side up)
- 50ml light cream
- 2 tbsp grated Parmesan
- 1 tbsp olive oil
- 1 clove garlic, minced
- Salt and pepper, to taste
- Fresh parsley, chopped (optional, for garnish)

1. Cook the spaghetti in salted boiling water according to package. Drain and set aside.
2. In a pan, heat olive oil over medium heat and sauté garlic until fragrant.
3. Stir in the light cream and Parmesan (if using), and simmer for 2 minutes. Add salt and pepper to taste.
4. Toss the cooked spaghetti in the cream sauce until well coated.
5. Plate the spaghetti, then top with fried eggs and bacon. Garnish with parsley if desired.

SPICY EGG AND COUSCOUS BOWL

DF, SF, NF

PREP TIME: 10 mins **COOK TIME:** 20 mins **SERVINGS:** 2

CALORIES: 340 | CARBS: 38G | FAT: 14G | PROTEIN: 15G | FIBER: 6G

- 2 large eggs
- 1 cup cooked couscous
- ½ cup cherry tomatoes, halved
- ¼ cup chopped cucumber
- ¼ cup cooked chickpeas
- 2 tbsp harissa paste
- 1 tbsp olive oil
- ¼ tsp smoked paprika
- 1 tbsp chopped parsley

1. Heat olive oil in a pan, stir in harissa paste and smoked paprika, and cook for 1 minute.
2. Add couscous, chickpeas, and tomatoes. Stir and cook for 5 minutes.
3. Fry eggs in a separate pan. Serve couscous topped with fried eggs, cucumber, and parsley.

EGG AND TEFF PORRIDGE WITH SPICES AND NUTS

GF, DF, SF

PREP TIME: 10 mins **COOK TIME:** 20 mins **SERVINGS:** 2

CALORIES: 300 | CARBS: 34G | FAT: 10G | PROTEIN: 12G | FIBER: 4G

- 1 cup cooked teff
- 1 boiled egg, diced
- 1 tbsp chopped pistachios
- ¼ tsp ground cardamom
- 1 tbsp maple syrup

1. In a saucepan, warm the cooked teff over low heat, stirring occasionally.
2. Stir in the maple syrup and ground cardamom until fully incorporated.
3. Spoon the teff into serving bowls and top with the chopped pistachios and diced boiled egg.
4. Serve warm for a hearty, protein-rich breakfast or snack.

SORGHUM EGG STIR-FRY

GF, DF, SF, NF

PREP TIME: 10 mins **COOK TIME:** 20 mins **SERVINGS:** 2

CALORIES: 310 | CARBS: 38G | FAT: 10G | PROTEIN: 13G | FIBER: 4G

- 1 cup cooked sorghum
- 2 large eggs
- ¼ cup diced zucchini
- ¼ tsp turmeric
- 1 tbsp coconut oil

1. Heat coconut oil and sauté zucchini for 3 minutes.
2. Add sorghum and turmeric, mixing well.
3. Push sorghum to the side, scramble eggs, then combine everything.

CREAMY POLENTA WITH SOFT-BOILED EGGS

GF, DF, SF, NF

PREP TIME: 10 mins **COOK TIME:** 20 mins **SERVINGS:** 2

CALORIES: 320 | CARBS: 28G | FAT: 14G | PROTEIN: 15G | FIBER: 2G

- 1 cup cooked polenta
- 2 soft-boiled eggs
- ¼ cup grated parmesan cheese
- ¼ cup sautéed kale
- 1 tbsp butter
- ¼ tsp black pepper

1. Warm the polenta with butter and Parmesan cheese over low heat.
2. Top with sautéed kale and halved soft-boiled eggs. Sprinkle black pepper before serving.

PARSLEY BULGUR TABBOULEH

DF, SF, NF

PREP TIME: 10 mins **COOK TIME:** 15 mins **SERVINGS:** 2

CALORIES: 310 | CARBS: 38G | FAT: 10G | PROTEIN: 13G | FIBER: 4G

- 1 cup cooked bulgur
- 2 boiled eggs, diced
- 1/4 cup chopped parsley
- 1/4 cup diced tomatoes
- 1 tbsp olive oil
- 1 tbsp lemon juice

1. In a large bowl, combine the cooked bulgur, diced boiled eggs, chopped parsley, and diced tomatoes.
2. Drizzle the mixture with olive oil and fresh lemon juice.
3. Gently toss until everything is evenly coated.
4. Serve immediately as a light and refreshing dish.

SHAKSHUKA WITH LENTILS AND HERBS

GF, DF, SF, NF

PREP TIME: 10 mins **COOK TIME:** 20 mins **SERVINGS:** 2

CALORIES: 290 | CARBS: 24G | FAT: 10G | PROTEIN: 18G | FIBER: 6G

- 2 large eggs
- ½ cup cooked lentils
- ½ cup crushed tomatoes
- ¼ cup diced onions
- ¼ tsp smoked paprika
- 1 tbsp olive oil
- Fresh cilantro for garnish

1. Heat olive oil and sauté onions for 3 minutes. Add lentils, tomatoes, and paprika, then simmer for 5 minutes.
2. Create small wells in the mixture and crack eggs into them. Cover and cook until eggs are set.
3. Garnish with cilantro before serving.

FLUFFY OMELETTE RICE

GF, NF,
DF (IF USING GLUTEN AND DF VERSION)

PREP TIME: 10 mins **COOK TIME:** 15 mins **SERVINGS:** 4

CALORIES: 450 KCAL | PROTEIN: 15G | CARBS: 35G | FAT: 15G | FIBER: 2G

- 2 cups cooked rice (preferably cold)
- 1 small carrot, finely diced
- ¼ cup peas or corn (optional)
- ½ onion, finely chopped
- 1 tbsp oil (vegetable or olive oil)
- 2 tbsp ketchup (plus extra for garnish)
- 2 tsp soy sauce (or tamari for gluten-free)
- 2 tbsp milk (or dairy-free alternative)
- Salt and pepper, to taste
- Chopped chives or parsley for garnish

1. Sauté onion, carrot, and peas or corn in oil until soft.
2. Stir in rice, ketchup, and soy sauce; season with salt and pepper. Set aside.
3. Whisk eggs, milk, and a pinch of salt.
4. Cook half the eggs in a non-stick pan until mostly set. Add half the rice, fold the omelette, and plate. Repeat.
5. Top with homemade ketchup and garnish with chives or parsley.

EGG AND BUCKWHEAT PORRIDGE

GF, DF, SF

PREP TIME: 5 mins **COOK TIME:** 15 mins **SERVINGS:** 2

CALORIES: 350 KCAL | PROTEIN: 16G | CARBS: 30G | FAT: 18G | FIBER: 6G

- ½ cup buckwheat groats
- 2 eggs (scrambled or fried)
- 1 tsp olive oil
- ½ avocado, sliced
- 1 tbsp chia seeds or hemp seeds
- Salt and pepper to taste
- Fresh herbs like cilantro or parsley (for garnish)

1. Cook the buckwheat in water for 10–12 minutes until tender.
2. In a separate pan, scramble or fry the eggs in olive oil.
3. Serve the cooked buckwheat topped with eggs, avocado slices, and a sprinkle of chia or hemp seeds.
4. Garnish with fresh herbs and season with salt and pepper to taste.

EGG AND BARLEY PILAF WITH DRIED FRUITS

DF, SF

PREP TIME: 10 mins **COOK TIME:** 20 mins **SERVINGS:** 2
CALORIES: 320 | CARBS: 38G | FAT: 10G | PROTEIN: 13G | FIBER: 5G

- 1 cup cooked barley
- 2 boiled eggs, diced
- 1 tbsp raisins
- 1 tbsp chopped almonds
- ¼ tsp cinnamon

1. In a large mixing bowl, combine the cooked barley with raisins, chopped almonds, and ground cinnamon. Toss gently to mix well.
2. Divide the mixture into serving bowls and top with the diced boiled eggs.
3. Serve warm or at room temperature for a comforting, nutritious meal.

MUSHROOM AND SCRAMBLED BARLEY RISOTTO

DF, SF, NF

PREP TIME: 10 mins **COOK TIME:** 20 mins **SERVINGS:** 2
CALORIES: 300 | CARBS: 35G | FAT: 10G | PROTEIN: 14G | FIBER: 5G

- 1 cup cooked barley
- 2 large eggs
- ½ cup diced mushrooms
- ¼ cup chopped onion
- 1 tbsp olive oil
- ¼ tsp thyme
- ¼ tsp black pepper

1. Heat olive oil in a skillet and sauté onions and mushrooms for 5 minutes.
2. Add barley, thyme, and black pepper. Stir well and cook for 10 minutes.
3. Scramble eggs separately and mix into the barley before serving.

MOROCCAN SCRAMBLED EGGS WITH CRUSTY BREAD

GF, DF

PREP TIME: 5 mins **COOK TIME:** 10 mins **SERVINGS:** 2
CALORIES: 300 KCAL | PROTEIN: 22G | CARBS: 18G | FAT: 18G | FIBER: 3G

- 4 eggs
- 1 tbsp olive oil
- ¼ tsp turmeric
- ¼ tsp cumin
- ¼ cup chopped tomatoes (or diced cherry tomatoes)
- Salt and pepper to taste
- Fresh cilantro or parsley (for garnish)
- 2 slices of crusty bread

1. Heat olive oil in a skillet over medium heat.
2. Crack the eggs directly into the skillet and stir with turmeric, cumin, salt, and pepper to scramble.
3. Add the chopped tomatoes and cook until eggs are fluffy and tomatoes soften slightly.
4. Garnish with fresh cilantro or parsley and serve with a slice of crusty bread on the side.

SPINACH AND FETA EGG MUFFINS

GF, V, SF, NF

PREP TIME: 10 mins **COOK TIME:** 15 mins **SERVINGS:** 4
CALORIES: 120 KCAL | PROTEIN: 9G | CARBS: 3G | FAT: 8G | FIBER: 1G

- 4 large eggs
- 1 cup fresh spinach, chopped
- ¼ cup feta cheese, crumbled
- ¼ cup diced bell pepper
- ¼ tsp dried oregano
- ¼ tsp garlic powder
- Salt and pepper to taste
- Olive oil spray
- Fresh herbs like parsley or basil (for garnish)

1. Preheat the oven to 350°F (175°C) and lightly spray a muffin tin with olive oil.
2. In a bowl, whisk together eggs, spinach, bell pepper, feta, oregano, garlic powder, salt, and pepper.
3. Pour the mixture evenly into the muffin tin.
4. Bake for 15 minutes, or until the eggs are set and slightly golden on top.
5. Garnish with fresh herbs before serving.

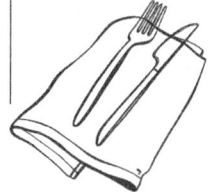

Scan this QR code to download recipes with vibrant, full-color photos,
'A Handbook of 100 Classic Anti-Inflammatory Recipes with Full Colored Pictures'

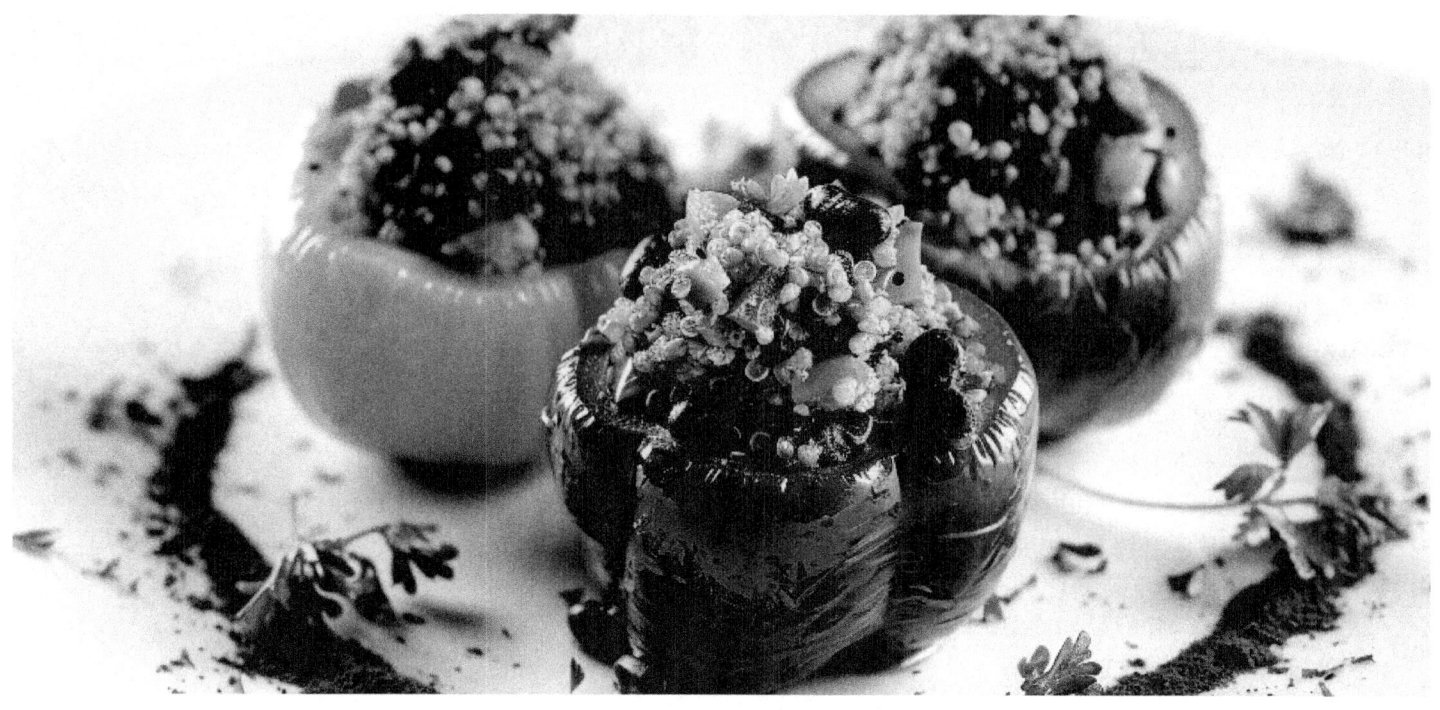

CHAPTER 11
VEGETABLES

"Let a medley of vegetables fill your plate - a key building block for longevity."

Vegetable recipes focus on including nutrient-dense vegetables like leafy greens, cruciferous vegetables (such as broccoli, kale, and cauliflower), and root vegetables (like sweet potatoes and beets).

These veggies are rich in antioxidants, fiber, vitamins (like C and K), and phytonutrients that help lower inflammation by neutralizing free radicals and reducing oxidative stress.

Regular consumption of these foods may help reduce the risk of chronic conditions such as heart disease, diabetes, and arthritis.

TIPS:

- **FATS:** Use anti-inflammatory fats like olive oil, avocado, and nuts to help absorb fat-soluble vitamins.

- **STORAGE:** Store prepared vegetable dishes in an airtight container in the refrigerator for up to 3-4 days.

- **FREEZE FOR LONGEVITY:** Some vegetable-based dishes (like stews) can be frozen for up to 3 months.

STUFFED ACORN SQUASH WITH LENTILS AND POMEGRANATE

VG, GF, DF, SF, V

PREP TIME: 5 mins **COOK TIME:** 25 mins **SERVINGS:** 2

CALORIES: 300 | CARBS: 50G | FAT: 10G | PROTEIN: 12G | FIBER: 10G

- 2 acorn squashes, halved and seeded
- ½ cup cooked lentils
- ¼ cup pomegranate seeds
- 1 tbsp olive oil
- 1 tsp ground cumin
- 1 tsp cinnamon
- Salt and pepper to taste
- Fresh parsley for garnish

1. Preheat oven to 200°C (400°F). Brush squash halves with olive oil, season with cumin, cinnamon, salt, and pepper. Roast for 25 minutes.
2. In a bowl, mix cooked lentils with pomegranate seeds.
3. Once squash is tender, stuff with lentil mixture and garnish with parsley. Serve warm.

CAULIFLOWER AND CHICKPEA CURRY

VG, GF, SF, NF, V

PREP TIME: 5 mins **COOK TIME:** 25 mins **SERVINGS:** 2

CALORIES: 320 | CARBS: 35G | FAT: 16G | PROTEIN: 10G | FIBER: 12G

- 1 small cauliflower, cut into florets
- 1 cup cooked chickpeas
- 1 tbsp curry powder
- 1 tsp cumin
- 1 tsp paprika
- 1 tbsp olive oil
- 1 can (400ml) coconut milk
- 1 tbsp tomato paste
- Salt and pepper to taste

1. Fresh cilantro for garnish
2. Heat olive oil in a pan and sauté cauliflower florets until slightly tender.
3. Add curry powder, cumin, paprika, and salt. Stir for 1–2 minutes.
4. Pour in coconut milk and tomato paste. Stir, cover, and simmer for 15 minutes.
5. Add cooked chickpeas and cook for an additional 5 minutes.
6. Garnish with fresh cilantro and serve.

ROASTED TURNIPS AND CARROTS WITH MUSTARD

VG, GF, DF, SF, NF, V

PREP TIME: 10 mins **COOK TIME:** 20 mins **SERVINGS:** 2

CALORIES: 180 | CARBS: 35G | FAT: 8G | PROTEIN: 3G | FIBER: 8G

- 3 medium turnips, peeled and diced
- 3 medium carrots, peeled and diced
- 1 tbsp olive oil
- 1 tbsp Dijon mustard
- 1 tsp thyme
- Salt and pepper to taste

1. Preheat oven to 200°C (400°F).
2. Toss turnips and carrots with olive oil, Dijon mustard, thyme, salt, and pepper.
3. Roast for 20 minutes, stirring halfway through, until golden and tender.
4. Serve warm.

SAUTEED BELGIUM ENDIVES WITH ORANGES

VG, GF, DF, V

PREP TIME: 10 mins **COOK TIME:** 10 mins **SERVINGS:** 2

CALORIES: 180 | CARBS: 24G | FAT: 10G | PROTEIN: 2G | FIBER: 6G

- 4 belgian endives, sliced
- 2 oranges, peeled and segmented
- 1 tbsp olive oil
- 1 tsp honey
- Salt and pepper to taste

1. Heat olive oil in a pan. Add endive slices and sauté for 5-7 minutes until soft.
2. Drizzle with honey and toss with orange segments.
3. Season with salt and pepper, and serve warm.

STUFFED BELL PEPPERS WITH QUINOA AND BLACK BEANS

GF, VG, SF, V

PREP TIME: 10 mins **COOK TIME:** 20 mins **SERVINGS:** 2

CALORIES: 220 KCAL | PROTEIN: 8G | CARBS: 35G | FAT: 7G | FIBER: 10G

- 2 large bell peppers, halved and seeds removed
- 1 cup cooked quinoa
- ½ cup black beans, cooked
- 1 tbsp olive oil
- ¼ tsp cumin
- ¼ tsp chili powder
- Salt and pepper to taste
- Fresh cilantro (for garnish)

4. Preheat the oven to 375°F (190°C).
5. In a bowl, mix the cooked quinoa, black beans, olive oil, cumin, chili powder, salt, and pepper.
6. Stuff the bell pepper halves with the quinoa mixture and place them on a baking sheet.
7. Bake for 20 minutes, or until the peppers are tender. Garnish with fresh cilantro before serving.

CABBAGE STIR-FRY WITH GINGER AND CARROTS

GF, VG, SF, V

PREP TIME: 10 mins **COOK TIME:** 10 mins **SERVINGS:** 2

CALORIES: 100 KCAL | PROTEIN: 2G | CARBS: 10G | FAT: 7G | FIBER: 3G

- 2 cups cabbage, shredded
- 1 carrot, julienned
- 1 tbsp olive oil
- ½ tsp grated ginger
- ¼ tsp sesame seeds
- Salt and pepper to taste
- Red chili (optional)
- A splash of tamari or soy sauce for extra flavor (optional)

1. Heat olive oil in a pan over medium heat, then sauté the grated ginger and carrots for 2 minutes until fragrant.
2. Add the shredded cabbage and stir-fry for an additional 5 minutes until tender.
3. Season with salt, pepper, and a sprinkle of sesame seeds for added flavor.

ROASTED ROOT VEGETABLE MEDLEY WITH HERBS

VG, GF, DF, SF, NF, V

PREP TIME: 10 mins **COOK TIME:** 20 mins **SERVINGS:** 2

CALORIES: 210 | CARBS: 40G | FAT: 9G | PROTEIN: 2G | FIBER: 7G

- 1 cup diced carrots
- 1 cup diced parsnips
- 1 cup diced sweet potatoes
- 1 tbsp olive oil
- 1 tsp rosemary
- 1 tsp thyme
- ½ tsp garlic powder
- Salt and pepper to taste

1. Preheat oven to 200°C (400°F).
2. In a large bowl, toss the diced carrots, parsnips, and sweet potatoes with olive oil, rosemary, thyme, garlic powder, salt, and pepper until evenly coated.
3. Spread the vegetables in a single layer on a baking sheet.
4. Roast in the oven for 20 minutes, or until the vegetables are tender and lightly caramelized, stirring halfway through.
5. Remove from the oven and serve warm.

BUTTERNUT SQUASH AND BRUSSELS SPROUTS WITH MAPLE-DIJON GLAZE

VG, GF, SF, NF, V

PREP TIME: 10 mins **COOK TIME:** 20 mins **SERVINGS:** 2

CALORIES: 220 | CARBS: 35G | FAT: 10G | PROTEIN: 5G | FIBER: 9G

- 1 small butternut squash, peeled and diced
- 1 cup Brussels sprouts, halved
- 1 tbsp olive oil
- 1 tbsp maple syrup
- 1 tbsp Dijon mustard
- 1 tsp fresh thyme
- Salt and pepper to taste

1. Preheat oven to 200°C (400°F).
2. Toss butternut squash and Brussels sprouts in olive oil, salt, and pepper.
3. Roast on a baking sheet for 20 minutes, stirring halfway through.
4. In a small bowl, whisk together maple syrup, Dijon mustard, and thyme.
5. Drizzle glaze over roasted vegetables and toss. Serve warm.

KOREAN-STYLE TOFU AND VEGETABLES WITH GINGER GARLIC SAUCE

VG, GF, DF, V

PREP TIME: 10 mins **COOK TIME:** 15 mins **SERVINGS:** 2

CALORIES: 290 | CARBS: 15G | FAT: 22G | PROTEIN: 18G | FIBER: 5G

- 200g firm tofu, pressed and cubed
- 1 red bell pepper, julienned
- 1 cup baby spinach
- ½ cup mushrooms, sliced
- 2 tbsp soy sauce (or tamari for GF)
- 1 tbsp sesame oil
- 1 tbsp rice vinegar
- 1 tsp gochujang (Korean chili paste)
- 1 tbsp fresh ginger, minced
- 2 cloves garlic, minced
- 1 tbsp sesame seeds
- 2 tbsp chopped green onions

1. Heat sesame oil in a pan over medium heat. Add tofu cubes and sauté until golden and crispy, about 5–7 minutes.
2. Remove tofu and set aside. In the same pan, sauté the garlic, ginger, and vegetables until tender.
3. In a bowl, whisk together soy sauce, rice vinegar, and gochujang. Pour over the cooked vegetables and tofu, toss to coat.
4. Garnish with sesame seeds and green onions. Serve immediately.

STEWED VEGETABLE WITH TOFU AND MUSHROOMS

GF, VG, SF (OPTIONAL), V

PREP TIME: 10 mins **COOK TIME:** 20 mins **SERVINGS:** 2

CALORIES: 120 KCAL | PROTEIN: 7G | CARBS: 10G | FAT: 5G | FIBER: 4G

- 1 cup napa cabbage, chopped
- 1 cup bok choy, chopped
- ½ cup shiitake mushrooms, sliced
- ½ cup daikon radish, sliced
- ½ cup tofu, cubed (or tempeh for soy-free)
- 1 tsp sesame oil
- 1 clove garlic, minced
- ½ tsp grated ginger
- 3 cups vegetable broth
- 1 tbsp tamari (or coconut aminos for soy-free)
- ¼ tsp white pepper or chili flakes

1. Heat sesame oil in a large pot over medium heat. Add garlic and ginger, sautéing until fragrant (about 1 minute).
2. Add shiitake mushrooms and daikon radish. Stir-fry for 2-3 minutes.
3. Add vegetable broth and tamari. Bring to a gentle boil.
4. Add napa cabbage, bok choy, and tofu cubes. Lower the heat and simmer for 10 minutes until vegetables are tender.
5. Season with white pepper or chili flakes if desired. Serve hot.

GARLIC BUTTER ASPARAGUS WITH LEMON ZEST

VG, GF, SF, NF, V

PREP TIME: 5 mins **COOK TIME:** 10 mins **SERVINGS:** 2

CALORIES: 120 | CARBS: 8G | FAT: 10G | PROTEIN: 3G | FIBER: 4G

- 1 bunch asparagus, trimmed
- 1 tbsp butter
- 2 cloves garlic, minced
- Zest of 1 lemon
- Salt and pepper to taste

1. Heat butter in a skillet over medium heat.
2. Add garlic and sauté for 1 minute until fragrant.
3. Add asparagus, salt, and pepper. Cook for 5–7 minutes until tender.
4. Remove from heat, sprinkle with lemon zest, and serve.

CRISPY BAKED ARTICHOKE HEARTS

VG, GF, SF, NF, V

PREP TIME: 10 mins **COOK TIME:** 20 mins **SERVINGS:** 2

CALORIES: 220 | CARBS: 16G | FAT: 14G | PROTEIN: 6G | FIBER: 6G

- 1 can artichoke hearts, drained and halved
- 1 tbsp olive oil
- ¼ cup breadcrumbs
- 1 tbsp Parmesan cheese
- Salt and pepper to taste

1. Preheat oven to 200°C (400°F).
2. Toss artichoke hearts in olive oil, breadcrumbs, Parmesan, salt, and pepper.
3. Bake for 20 minutes until crispy and golden. Serve warm.

TURMERIC ROASTED CAULIFLOWER

GF, V, SF, NF, VG

PREP TIME: 10 mins **COOK TIME:** 20 mins **SERVINGS:** 4

CALORIES: 110 KCAL | PROTEIN: 4G | CARBS: 10G | FAT: 7G | FIBER: 3G

- 1 large head of cauliflower, cut into florets
- 2 tbsp olive oil
- 1 tsp turmeric
- ½ tsp garlic powder
- ¼ tsp cumin
- Salt and pepper to taste
- Fresh cilantro, chopped (for garnish)

1. Preheat the oven to 400°F (200°C).
2. In a large bowl, toss cauliflower florets with olive oil, turmeric, garlic powder, cumin, salt, and pepper.
3. Spread the cauliflower on a baking sheet and roast for 20 minutes until golden brown and tender.
4. Garnish with fresh cilantro before serving.

GINGER-GARLIC SAUTÉED SPINACH

GF, VG, SF, NF, V

PREP TIME: 5 mins **COOK TIME:** 5 mins **SERVINGS:** 2

CALORIES: 90 KCAL | PROTEIN: 3G | CARBS: 5G | FAT: 7G | FIBER: 2G

- 4 cups fresh spinach
- 1 tbsp olive oil
- 1 garlic clove, minced
- ½ tsp grated ginger
- ¼ tsp red pepper flakes
- Salt and pepper to taste
- Lemon juice

1. Heat olive oil in a pan over medium heat, add minced garlic, grated ginger, and red pepper flakes, sauté for 30 seconds until fragrant.
2. Add the spinach and cook until wilted, about 2-3 minutes, stirring occasionally.
3. Season with salt and pepper to taste, and finish with a squeeze of lemon juice.

HEARTY VEGETABLE STEW

GF, VG, SF, NF, DF, V

PREP TIME: 10 mins **COOK TIME:** 20 mins **SERVINGS:** 2

CALORIES: 190 KCAL | PROTEIN: 5G | CARBS: 28G | FAT: 5G | FIBER: 6G

- 1 tbsp olive oil
- 1 medium onion, diced
- 2 garlic cloves, minced
- 2 medium carrots, sliced
- 1 medium sweet potato, cubed
- 1 cup green peas (fresh or frozen)
- 1 can (400g) diced tomatoes
- 2 cups vegetable broth
- ½ brinjal sliced
- 1 tsp smoked paprika
- ½ tsp ground cumin
- ¼ tsp chili flakes (optional)
- Salt and pepper to taste
- Fresh parsley or cilantro for garnish

1. Heat olive oil in a pot over medium heat.
2. Sauté onions and garlic until softened (about 2 minutes).
3. Add carrots, sweet potato, brinjal, smoked paprika, cumin, and chili flakes. Stir and cook for 3 minutes.
4. Pour in diced tomatoes and vegetable broth. Bring to a boil, then reduce heat to simmer for 15 minutes, or until vegetables are tender.
5. Add green peas and cook for another 2 minutes. Adjust seasoning with salt and pepper.
6. Serve warm and garnish with fresh parsley or cilantro.

GRILLED ZUCCHINI AND EGGPLANT WITH LEMON TAHINI SAUCE

GF, VG, SF, NF, V

PREP TIME: 10 mins **COOK TIME:** 15 mins **SERVINGS:** 4

CALORIES: 150 KCAL | PROTEIN: 3G | CARBS: 10G | FAT: 11G | FIBER: 4G

- 2 zucchinis, sliced lengthwise
- 1 eggplant, sliced lengthwise
- 2 tbsp olive oil
- 2 tbsp tahini
- 1 tbsp lemon juice
- 1 garlic clove, minced
- ¼ tsp cumin
- Salt and pepper to taste
- Fresh parsley or cilantro (for garnish)

1. Preheat the grill to medium heat.
2. Brush the zucchini and eggplant slices with olive oil, and season with salt, pepper, and cumin.
3. Grill the vegetables for 3-4 minutes on each side until grill marks appear and they are tender.
4. In a small bowl, mix tahini, lemon juice, minced garlic, and a bit of water to thin the sauce to your desired consistency.
5. Drizzle the lemon tahini sauce over the grilled vegetables and garnish with fresh parsley or cilantro before serving.

CARAMELIZED ANTI-INFLAMMATORY VEGETABLES

GF, VG, SF, NF, DF, V

PREP TIME: 5 mins **COOK TIME:** 25 mins **SERVINGS:** 2

CALORIES: 150 KCAL | PROTEIN: 5G | CARBS: 15G | FAT: 7G | FIBER: 5G

- 1 cup broccoli florets
- 1 cup cauliflower florets
- ½ cup red onion, sliced
- 1 small carrot, sliced
- 1 tbsp olive oil
- ½ tsp garlic powder
- ¼ tsp smoked paprika
- Salt and pepper to taste

1. Preheat oven to 400°F (200°C).
2. Toss broccoli, cauliflower, red onion, and carrot in a bowl with olive oil, garlic powder, smoked paprika, salt, and pepper.
3. Spread the vegetables evenly on a parchment-lined baking sheet.
4. Roast for 20-25 minutes, flipping halfway through, until tender and slightly caramelized.
5. Serve warm as a side dish or enjoy as a light main meal.

ZUCCHINI NOODLES WITH PESTO

GF, VG, SF, NF, V

PREP TIME: 10 mins **COOK TIME:** 5 mins **SERVINGS:** 2

CALORIES: 200 KCAL | PROTEIN: 4G | CARBS: 8G | FAT: 18G | FIBER: 3G

- 2 medium zucchinis, spiralized
- 2 tbsp pesto (store-bought or homemade)
- 1 tbsp olive oil
- ¼ tsp red pepper flakes
- Cherry tomatoes, halved
- Fresh basil leaves (for garnish)

1. Wash the zucchinis thoroughly and trim off both ends. Using a spiralizer, create long, thin noodle-like strands.
2. Heat olive oil in a pan over medium heat and sauté zucchini noodles for 3–4 minutes until just tender.
3. Remove from heat and toss with pesto and cherry tomatoes.
4. Garnish with fresh basil leaves and red pepper flakes for a touch of heat.

SPICY SWEET POTATO FRIES

GF, VG, SF, NF, V

PREP TIME: 5 mins **COOK TIME:** 20 mins **SERVINGS:** 2

CALORIES: 180 KCAL | PROTEIN: 3G | CARBS: 28G | FAT: 7G | FIBER: 5G

- 2 medium sweet potatoes, cut into fries
- 1 tbsp olive oil
- ½ tsp chili powder
- ¼ tsp garlic powder
- ¼ tsp paprika
- Salt and pepper to taste
- Fresh parsley (for garnish)

1. Preheat the oven to 425°F (220°C).
2. Toss the sweet potato fries with olive oil, chili powder, garlic powder, paprika, salt, and pepper.
3. Spread the fries on a baking sheet in a single layer and roast for 20 minutes, flipping halfway through.
4. Garnish with fresh parsley before serving.

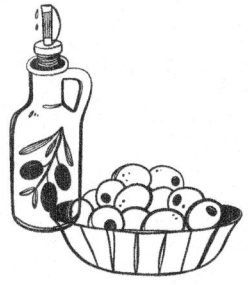

ROASTED PARSNIPS WITH LIME AND CILANTRO

VG, GF, DF, SF, NF, V

PREP TIME: 10 mins **COOK TIME:** 20 mins **SERVINGS:** 2

CALORIES: 220 | CARBS: 40G | FAT: 8G | PROTEIN: 3G | FIBER: 7G

- 3 medium parsnips, peeled and cut into wedges
- 1 tbsp olive oil
- 1 tsp smoked paprika
- ½ tsp chili powder
- Juice of 1 lime
- 2 tbsp fresh cilantro, chopped
- Salt and pepper to taste

1. Preheat oven to 200°C (400°F).
2. Toss parsnip wedges with olive oil, smoked paprika, chili powder, salt, and pepper.
3. Roast for 20 minutes, flipping halfway, until golden and tender.
4. Drizzle with lime juice and garnish with cilantro. Serve warm.

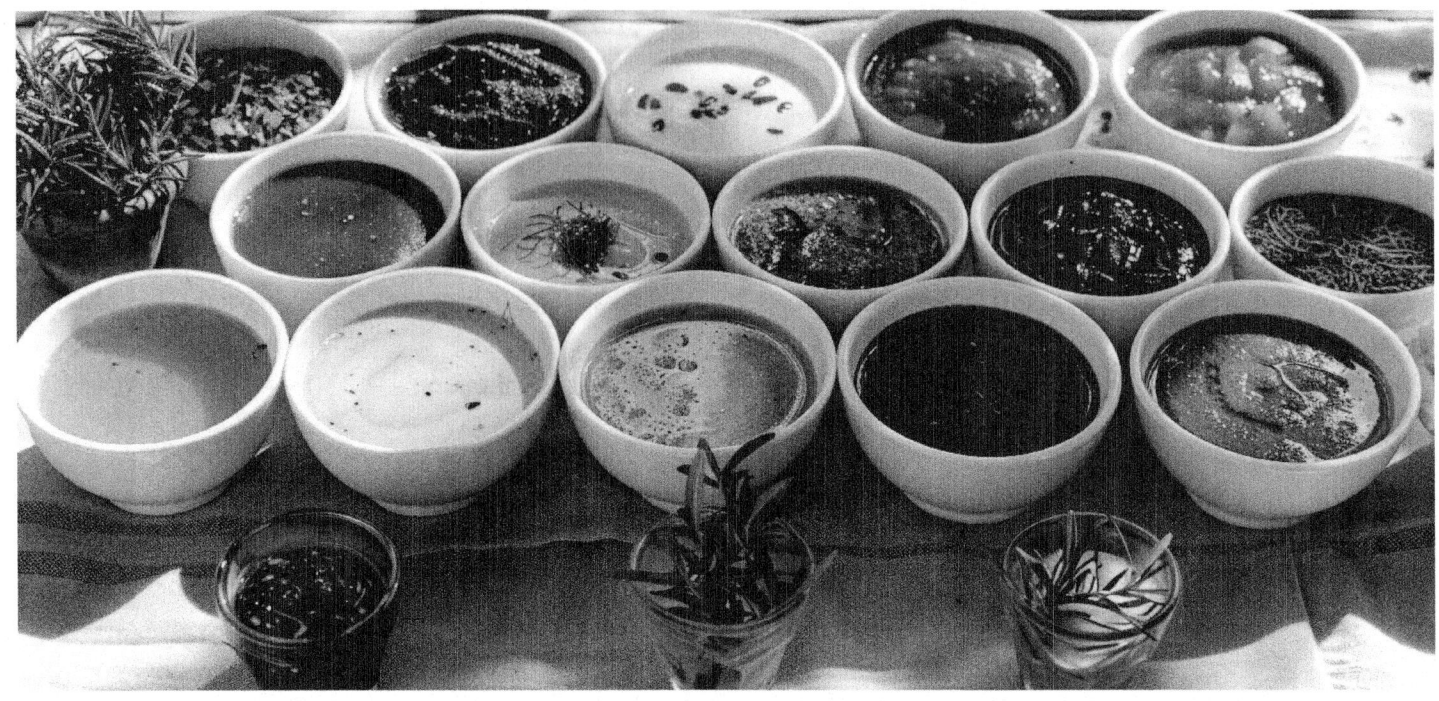

CHAPTER 12

SAUCES, CONDIMENTS AND DRESSINGS

"Spice it up with healing flavors to tease your palate and reawaken your health."

Homemade sauces, condiments, and dressings omit the need for store-bought options, which are often filled with additives and preservatives. They're much healthier and quick to prepare!

These anti-inflammatory recipes are loaded with ingredients like apple cider vinegar, turmeric, ginger, garlic, lemon, and olive oil. These are rich in antioxidants, healthy fats, and inflammation-fighting compounds.

They'll not only elevate your dishes but also promote gut health, support heart function, and help reduce chronic inflammation.

TIPS:

- **OILS:** Use cold-pressed olive oil and organic vinegars to ensure maximum health benefits.

- **AVOID REFINED SUGARS:** Opt for honey or maple syrup as natural sweeteners.

- **STORAGE:** Store homemade sauces and dressings in airtight containers in the refrigerator for up to 5 days.

BEETROOT CASHEW SAUCE

VG, GF, DF, SF, V

PREP TIME: 5 mins **COOK TIME:** 0 min **SERVINGS:** 4

CALORIES: 75 | CARBS: 5G | FAT: 4G | PROTEIN: 2G | FIBER: 1G | SODIUM: 12MG

- ¼ cup cashews, soaked
- ½ cup cooked beetroot, diced
- 1 tbsp lemon juice
- 2 tbsp water
- 1 clove garlic
- ½ tsp olive oil
- Pinch of salt and black pepper, to taste

1. In a blender or food processor, combine soaked cashews, beetroot, lemon juice, water, and garlic. Blend until smooth and creamy.
2. Add olive oil, salt, and black pepper. Blend again briefly to incorporate.
3. Taste and adjust seasoning if needed, adding more lemon juice for tang or water for a thinner consistency.
4. Use as a pasta sauce, dip, or spread.

WALNUT PARSLEY PESTO

VG, GF, DF, SF, V

PREP TIME: 5 mins **COOK TIME:** 0 min **SERVINGS:** 4

CALORIES: 95 | CARBS: 2G | FAT: 8G | PROTEIN: 2G | FIBER: 1G | SODIUM: 5MG

- ¼ cup walnuts
- 1 tbsp olive oil
- 1 tbsp lemon juice
- ½ cup fresh parsley
- 2 tbsp water (adjust for consistency)
- 1 small garlic clove
- 1 tbsp nutritional yeast
- Pinch of salt and black pepper, to taste

1. In a blender or food processor, combine walnuts, olive oil, lemon juice, parsley, water, and garlic (if using). Blend until smooth and creamy.
2. Add nutritional yeast, salt, and black pepper. Blend again briefly to incorporate.
3. Adjust the consistency by adding more water, 1 tsp at a time, if needed. Taste and adjust seasoning as desired.

CREAMY BASIL AVOCADO SAUCE

VG, GF, DF, SF, NF, V

PREP TIME: 5 mins **COOK TIME:** 0 min **SERVINGS:** 4

CALORIES: 75 | CARBS: 3G | FAT: 6G | PROTEIN: 1G | FIBER: 2G | SODIUM: 8MG

- 1 ripe avocado, peeled and pitted
- 2 tbsp fresh basil leaves
- 1 tbsp lemon juice
- 2 tbsp water (adjust for consistency)
- 1 tsp olive oil
- 1 small garlic clove
- ½ tsp nutritional yeast
- Pinch of salt and black pepper, to taste

1. Combine avocado, basil, lemon juice, water, olive oil, and garlic (if using) in a blender or food processor. Blend until smooth and creamy.
2. Add nutritional yeast, salt, and black pepper. Blend again briefly to combine.
3. Taste and adjust seasoning if necessary, adding more water for a thinner consistency.
4. Use for salads, pasta, grain bowls, tacos, roasted vegetables, or as a spread for sandwiches and wraps.

RASPBERRY VINAIGRETTE

VG, GF, DF, SF, NF, V

PREP TIME: 5 mins **COOK TIME:** 0 min **SERVINGS:** 4

CALORIES: 42 | CARBS: 3G | FAT: 3G | PROTEIN: 0G | FIBER: 1G | SODIUM: 6MG

- ¼ cup fresh raspberries
- 1 tbsp balsamic vinegar
- 1 tsp honey (or maple syrup for a vegan option)
- 1 tbsp olive oil
- 2 tbsp water
- ¼ tsp Dijon mustard
- Pinch of salt and black pepper, to taste

1. Combine raspberries, balsamic vinegar, honey, olive oil, water, and Dijon mustard (if using) in a blender. Blend until smooth.
2. Taste and season with salt and black pepper as desired.
3. Strain through a fine mesh sieve if a smoother texture is preferred.
4. Drizzle over mixed greens, roasted vegetables, or use as a marinade. Store leftovers in the refrigerator for up to 3 days in an airtight container.

ZESTY CHIMICHURRI SAUCE

VG, GF, DF, SF, NF, V

PREP TIME: 5 mins **COOK TIME:** 0 min **SERVINGS:** 4

CALORIES: 85 | CARBS: 2G | FAT: 7G | PROTEIN: 1G | FIBER: 0G | SODIUM: 20MG

- 1 cup fresh parsley, finely chopped
- 2 tbsp fresh cilantro, finely chopped
- 1 tbsp red wine vinegar
- 2 tbsp olive oil
- 1 clove garlic, minced
- 1 tsp chili flakes
- 1 tsp lemon zest
- Pinch of salt and black pepper, to taste

1. In a bowl, combine parsley, cilantro (if using), red wine vinegar, and olive oil.
2. Stir in minced garlic, chili flakes, and lemon zest, mixing well.
3. Season with salt and pepper to taste.
4. Serve fresh as a topping for grilled veggies, protein, or salads. Refrigerate leftovers in an airtight container for up to 3 days.

POMEGRANTE MINT SAUCE

VG, GF, DF, SF, V

PREP TIME: 5 mins **COOK TIME:** 0 min **SERVINGS:** 4

CALORIES: 52 | CARBS: 7G | FAT: 3G | PROTEIN: 0G | FIBER: 1G | SODIUM: 10MG

- ½ cup pomegranate seeds
- 1 tbsp fresh mint, finely chopped
- 1 tbsp lemon juice
- 1 tsp honey (or maple syrup for vegan)
- 1 tbsp olive oil
- ¼ tsp ground cumin
- Pinch of salt

1. Blend pomegranate seeds, lemon juice, honey, and cumin (if using) in a blender until smooth.
2. Strain the mixture through a fine mesh sieve to remove the pulp.
3. Stir in olive oil, chopped mint, and a pinch of salt. Mix well.
4. Serve immediately as a dip, drizzle, or salad dressing. Store in an airtight container in the refrigerator for up to 3 days.

SESAME GINGER SAUCE

VG, GF, DF, NF, V

PREP TIME: 5 mins **COOK TIME:** 0 min **SERVINGS:** 4

CALORIES: 60 | CARBS: 2G | FAT: 5G | PROTEIN: 2G | FIBER: 1G | SODIUM: 150MG

- 2 tbsp tahini
- 1 tbsp soy sauce (or tamari for gluten-free)
- 1 tbsp rice vinegar
- 1 tsp fresh ginger, grated
- 1 tsp maple syrup or honey
- ½ tsp toasted sesame oil
- 1 tbsp water
- Pinch of chili flakes or a dash of hot sauce

1. In a small bowl, whisk together tahini, soy sauce, rice vinegar, grated ginger, and maple syrup or honey (if using).
2. Add toasted sesame oil and chili flakes for extra flavor, if desired.
3. Gradually whisk in water until the sauce reaches your preferred consistency.
4. Serve immediately as a dip, drizzle, or salad dressing. Store leftovers in an airtight container in the refrigerator for up to 3 days.

SPICY COCONUT SAUCE

VG, GF, DF, V

PREP TIME: 5 mins **COOK TIME:** 0 min **SERVINGS:** 4

CALORIES: 85 | CARBS: 6G | FAT: 6G | PROTEIN: 1G | FIBER: 0G | SODIUM: 20MG

- ½ cup coconut milk
- 1 tsp red curry paste
- 1 tsp lime juice
- 1 tbsp peanut butter (or almond butter)
- 1 tsp honey (or maple syrup for vegan)
- ½ tsp grated ginger
- ½ tsp soy sauce (or tamari for GF)
- Pinch of chili flakes or a dash of hot sauce

1. In a medium bowl, whisk together the coconut milk, red curry paste, peanut butter, and soy sauce until smooth.
2. Add lime juice, honey, grated ginger, and chili flakes (if using). Mix well to combine.
3. Taste and adjust seasoning as needed, adding more lime juice for tang or honey for sweetness.
4. Serve immediately as a dip, sauce, or dressing.

SWEET CHILLI DIPPING SAUCE

VG, GF, DF, SF, NF, V (OPTIONAL)
PREP TIME: 5 mins   **COOK TIME:** 5 mins   **SERVINGS:** 4
CALORIES: 42 | CARBS: 11G | FAT: 0G | PROTEIN: 0G | FIBER: 0G | SODIUM: 18MG

- 2 tbsp honey (or maple syrup for vegan)
- 1 tbsp rice vinegar
- 1 tsp chili flakes
- 1 tsp grated ginger
- 1 small garlic clove, minced
- 1 tbsp water
- 1 tsp cornstarch
- Pinch of salt

1. In a small saucepan, combine honey, rice vinegar, chili flakes, ginger, and garlic. Heat gently over medium-low.
2. In a separate bowl, dissolve cornstarch in water, then add the mixture to the saucepan.
3. Simmer for 3–5 minutes, stirring constantly, until the sauce thickens and becomes glossy.
4. Taste and adjust seasoning with a pinch of salt, if needed.
5. Remove from heat, let cool slightly, and serve as a dipping sauce or drizzle.

ALMOND BUTTER AND GINGER DIP

VG, GF, DF, V
PREP TIME: 5 mins   **COOK TIME:** 0 min   **SERVINGS:** 4
CALORIES: 35 | CARBS: 2G | FAT: 3G | PROTEIN: 1G | FIBER: 0G | SODIUM: 55MG

- 3 tbsp almond butter
- 1 tbsp soy sauce (or tamari for GF)
- 1 tbsp lime juice
- 1 tsp fresh ginger, grated
- 1 tsp maple syrup or honey
- ½ tsp garlic, minced or grated
- 1 tbsp water
- Pinch of chili flakes or a dash of hot sauce

1. In a small bowl, combine almond butter, soy sauce, lime juice, and maple syrup or honey if using.
2. Add grated ginger, garlic, and water, whisking until smooth and creamy.
3. Adjust consistency by adding more water, 1 tsp at a time, if needed.
4. Taste and adjust flavors, adding a pinch of chili flakes or a dash of hot sauce for heat, if desired.
5. Serve immediately as a dip for vegetables, a drizzle over salads, or as a sauce for noodle dishes.

CREAMY CASHEW GARLIC SAUCE

GF, VG, V
PREP TIME: 20 mins (plus cashew soaking time)
COOK TIME: 0 min   **SERVINGS:** 4
CALORIES: 120 KCAL | PROTEIN: 4G | CARBS: 8G | FAT: 9G | FIBER: 1G

- ½ cup raw cashews (soak in hot water for 20 minutes)
- 1 clove garlic
- 2 tbsp nutritional yeast
- 1 tbsp lemon juice
- ¼ cup water
- Salt to taste

1. Blend all until creamy and smooth. Add water as needed to achieve the desired consistency.
2. Adjust seasoning to taste, and serve as desired.

HOMEMADE TOMATO KETCHUP

GF, VG, V

PREP TIME: 5 mins **COOK TIME:** 20 mins **SERVINGS:** 4

CALORIES: 25 KCAL | PROTEIN: 5G | CARBS: 6G | FAT: 0G | FIBER: 1G

- 6 medium ripe tomatoes, chopped
- ¼ cup apple cider vinegar
- 3 tbsp sugar or a natural sweetener
- ½ tsp salt
- ¼ tsp ground black pepper
- ¼ tsp garlic powder
- ⅛ tsp ground cinnamon

1. Add chopped tomatoes to a medium-sized saucepan and cook over medium heat, stirring occasionally, until softened (about 10 minutes).
2. Blend the softened tomatoes in a blender or food processor until smooth. Pass the mixture through a sieve to remove any seeds or skin.
3. Return the strained tomato puree to the saucepan. Add apple cider vinegar, sugar, salt, black pepper, garlic powder, and cinnamon (if using).
4. Cook over low heat, stirring frequently, until the mixture thickens to a ketchup-like consistency (approximately 10 minutes).
5. Let the ketchup cool and transfer to a clean, airtight jar. Store in the refrigerator for up to two weeks.

TAMARIND SAUCE

VG, GF, DF, NF, V

PREP TIME: 5 mins **COOK TIME:** 0 min **SERVINGS:** 4

CALORIES: 75 | CARBS: 18G | FAT: 0G | PROTEIN: 0G | FIBER: 1G | SODIUM: 125MG

- 2 tbsp tamarind paste
- 2 tbsp honey (or maple syrup for vegan)
- 1 tbsp lime juice
- 1 tsp soy sauce (or tamari for gluten free)
- 1 clove garlic, minced
- ½ tsp grated ginger
- ½ tsp chili flakes
- ¼ tsp ground cumin
- 1 tbsp water

1. Combine tamarind paste, honey, lime juice, soy sauce, garlic, ginger, chili flakes, and cumin in a small saucepan.
2. Heat gently over low heat for 5–10 minutes, stirring occasionally, until the flavors meld. Add a splash of water if the sauce is too thick.
3. Taste and adjust sweetness or acidity as needed. Remove from heat and let it cool slightly before serving.
4. Use as a marinade or dipping sauce for grilled chicken, lamb, or pork.

LEMON-TURMERIC VINAIGRETTE

GF, NF, VG (IF USING MAPLE SYRUP), V (OPTIONAL)

PREP TIME: 5 mins **COOK TIME:** 0 min **SERVINGS:** 4

CALORIES: 100 KCAL | PROTEIN: 0G | CARBS: 2G | FAT: 10G | FIBER: 0G

- 2 tbsp lemon juice
- 1 tsp turmeric powder
- 1 tsp honey (or maple syrup for vegan)
- 3 tbsp olive oil
- 1 clove garlic, minced
- Salt & pepper to taste
- Optional: ¼ tsp black pepper

1. Whisk all together in a bowl until emulsified and smooth.
2. Adjust seasoning to taste and use as a dressing for salads, roasted veggies, or grain bowls.

GINGER-SOY DRESSING

GF (WITH TAMARI), NF, VG (IF USING MAPLE SYRUP), V

PREP TIME: 5 mins **COOK TIME:** 0 min **SERVINGS:** 4

CALORIES: 35 KCAL | PROTEIN: 1G | CARBS: 5G | FAT: 1G | FIBER: 0G

- 2 tbsp soy sauce (or tamari for gluten-free)
- 1 tbsp rice vinegar
- 1 tsp grated ginger
- 1 tsp sesame oil
- 1 tsp honey (or maple syrup for vegan)
- 1 clove garlic, minced
- Optional: ¼ tsp red pepper flakes

1. Mix all in a small bowl or jar. Shake well until combined.
2. Adjust seasoning to taste and serve over salads, steamed veggies, or as a marinade.

AVOCADO-CILANTRO SAUCE

GF, VG, NF, V

PREP TIME: 5 mins **COOK TIME:** 0 min **SERVINGS:** 4

CALORIES: 120 KCAL | PROTEIN: 1G | CARBS: 3G | FAT: 11G | FIBER: 3G

- 1 ripe avocado
- ¼ cup fresh cilantro
- 1 tbsp lime juice
- 2 tbsp olive oil
- Salt & pepper to taste
- Optional: 1 small garlic clove

1. Blend all until smooth. Add water as needed to achieve your desired consistency.
2. Adjust seasoning to taste and enjoy as a dip, dressing, or spread.

SPICY MANGO CHUTNEY

GF, NF, VG (IF USING MAPLE SYRUP), V

PREP TIME: 5 mins **COOK TIME:** 5-7 mins **SERVINGS:** 4

CALORIES: 70 KCAL | PROTEIN: 5G | CARBS: 18G | FAT: 5G | FIBER: 1G

- 1 ripe mango, chopped
- 1 tbsp apple cider vinegar
- ½ tsp chili powder
- 1 tsp grated ginger
- 1 tsp honey (or maple syrup for vegan)
- Optional: ¼ tsp turmeric powder

1. In a small saucepan, cook the mango, apple cider vinegar, ginger, chili powder, and turmeric (if using) over medium heat until the mango softens, about 5-7 minutes.
2. Blend the mixture for a smoother texture or leave it chunky for a more rustic feel. Adjust seasoning as desired.

GREEN GODDESS DRESSING

GF, VG, NF, V

PREP TIME: 10 mins **COOK TIME:** 0 min **SERVINGS:** 4

CALORIES: 90 KCAL | PROTEIN: 0G | CARBS: 2G | FAT: 9G | FIBER: 1G

- ½ cup parsley
- ¼ cup basil
- 1 clove garlic
- ¼ cup olive oil
- 2 tbsp apple cider vinegar
- 1 tbsp lemon juice
- Salt & pepper to taste

1. Blend all until smooth.
2. Adjust the seasoning as needed

GARLIC DILL SAUCE

VG, GF, SF, V

PREP TIME: 5 mins **COOK TIME:** 0 min **SERVINGS:** 4

CALORIES: 50 | CARBS: 3G | FAT: 2.5G | PROTEIN: 3G | FIBER: 0G | SODIUM: 80MG

- ½ cup plain Greek yogurt
- 1 tbsp lemon juice
- 1 clove garlic, minced
- 1 tbsp fresh dill, chopped
- 1 tsp honey
- ½ tsp Dijon mustard
- 1 tbsp olive oil
- ½ tsp onion powder
- Salt and black pepper to taste

1. Mix Greek yogurt, lemon juice, garlic, dill, honey, Dijon mustard, olive oil, onion powder, salt, and black pepper in a bowl until smooth.
2. Serve immediately or let it chill for at least 5 minutes to allow the flavors to meld together.
3. Pair with grilled meats, roasted vegetables, salads, wraps, and as a dip for pita or veggies.

TURMERIC-TAHINI DRESSING

GF, VG, NF, V

PREP TIME: 5 mins **COOK TIME:** 0 min **SERVINGS:** 4

CALORIES: 98 KCAL | PROTEIN: 3G | CARBS: 8G | FAT: 7G | FIBER: 2G

- ¼ cup tahini
- 1 tbsp lemon juice
- ½ tsp turmeric powder
- 1 clove garlic, minced
- 1 tbsp maple syrup
- ¼ cup water
- Pinch of salt & pepper
- Optional: ¼ tsp cumin

1. In a bowl, whisk together tahini, lemon juice, turmeric, minced garlic, maple syrup, salt, and pepper.
2. Gradually add water, whisking until smooth and the desired consistency is reached.

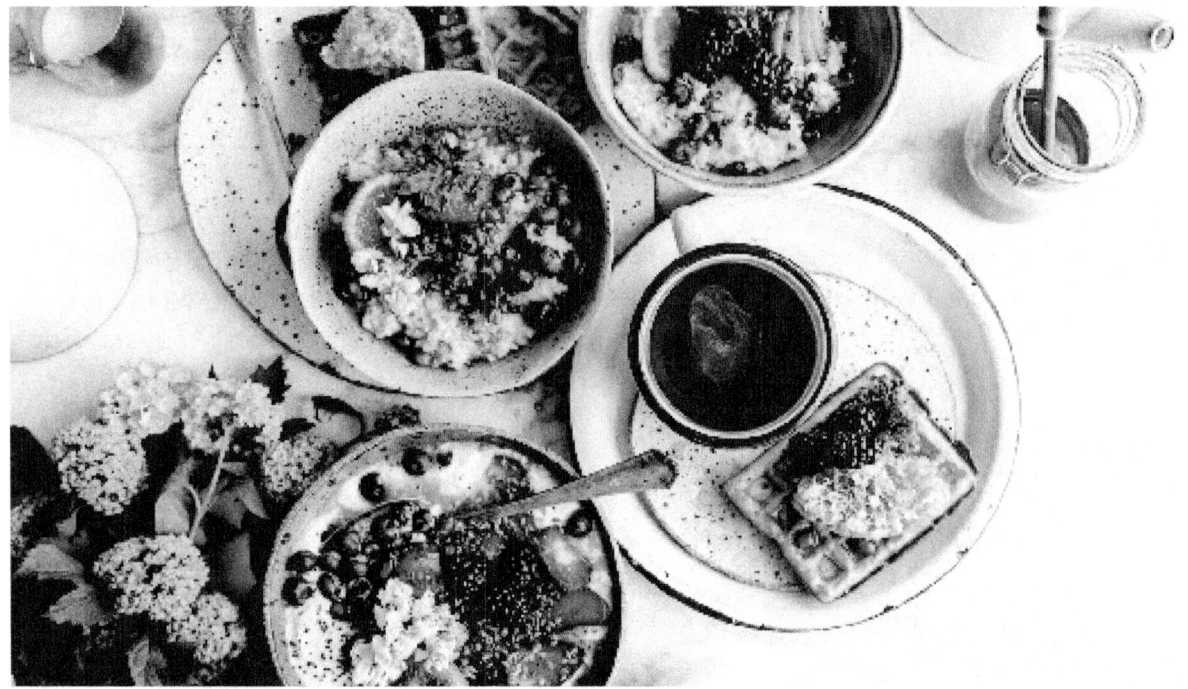

CHAPTER 13

SNACKS & QUICK BITES

"Roll with the punches - Small bites, big healing for stress-free days."

Injecting anti-inflammatory snacks into your diet is a powerful way to manage chronic inflammation, support a healthy immune system, and maintain overall well-being.

These snacks are packed with anti-inflammatory ingredients like omega-3 fatty acids, antioxidants, fiber, and phytonutrients, which help combat oxidative stress, lower inflammation markers, and improve metabolic health.

TIPS:

- **HEALTHY OPTIONS:** Opt for whole foods like fresh vegetables, fruits, nuts, seeds, and whole grains. Minimally processed snacks help maintain the anti-inflammatory benefits of the ingredients.

- **STORAGE:** Most anti-inflammatory snacks containing fresh fruits, veggies, nut butters, or yogurt should be stored in the fridge. For example, energy balls, hummus, and chia puddings can stay fresh in the refrigerator for up to 4-5 days.

WALNUTS AND DARK CHOCOLATE BITE

GF, VG, V

PREP TIME: 10 mins **CHILLING TIME:** 15-20 mins **SERVINGS:** 2
CALORIES: 240 KCAL | PROTEIN: 8G | CARBS: 20G | FAT: 16G | FIBER: 4G

- ½ cup walnuts
- ¼ cup dark chocolate chips (70% or higher cocoa)
- 1 tbsp dried cranberries
- 1 tbsp almond butter (or any nut/seed butter)
- 1 tbsp shredded coconut (unsweetened)
- ½ tsp cinnamon
- 1 tbsp pumpkin seeds
- Pinch of sea salt

1. Lightly chop the walnuts, dark chocolate chips, dried cranberries, and pumpkin seeds, or pulse them in a food processor until coarsely blended.
2. Transfer the mixture to a bowl, add shredded coconut, cinnamon, and a pinch of sea salt.
3. Add almond butter and mix until the stick together.
4. Scoop out small portions and roll them into bite-sized balls using your hands.
5. Place the bites on a plate or tray and refrigerate for 15–20 minutes to firm up.

AVOCADO-STUFFED SWEET POTATO BOATS

GF, VG, NF, DF, V

PREP TIME: 5 mins **COOK TIME:** 20 mins **SERVINGS:** 2
CALORIES: 210 KCAL | PROTEIN: 3G | CARBS: 36G | FAT: 13G | FIBER: 8G

- 1 medium sweet potato (halved lengthwise)
- ½ ripe avocado (mashed)
- 1 tbsp pomegranate seeds
- 1 tbsp fresh parsley or cilantro, chopped
- Pinch of sea salt and black pepper
- Optional: thinly sliced red chili for garnish

1. Preheat oven to 400°F (200°C).
2. Halve the sweet potato lengthwise and place it on a baking tray. Bake for 20–25 minutes or until tender.
3. Scoop and lightly mash the avocado with sea salt and black pepper.
4. Once the sweet potato halves are done, let them cool slightly, then top with mashed avocado.
5. Garnish with pomegranate seeds, fresh herbs, and optional chili slices for a pop of flavor and color.
6. Serve warm as a snack or light meal.

ROASTED PUMPKIN WITH THYME

GF, VG, NF, DF, V

PREP TIME: 5 mins **COOK TIME:** 25 mins **SERVINGS:** 4
CALORIES: 150 KCAL | PROTEIN: 2G | CARBS: 20G | FAT: 6G | FIBER: 4G

- 500g pumpkin, peeled and sliced into wedges
- 2 tbsp olive oil
- ½ tsp salt
- ¼ tsp black pepper
- ½ tsp paprika (optional)
- 1 tbsp fresh thyme leaves (or 1 tsp dried thyme)

1. Preheat the oven to 200°C (400°F).
2. In a large bowl, toss the pumpkin wedges with olive oil, salt, pepper, paprika, and thyme until evenly coated.
3. Spread the pumpkin wedges in a single layer on a baking tray lined with parchment paper.
4. Roast for 20-25 minutes, flipping halfway through, until the pumpkin is golden and tender.
5. Serve warm, garnished with extra thyme if desired.

ZUCCHINI PIZZA BITES

GF, SF, NF

PREP TIME: 5 mins **COOK TIME:** 10 mins **SERVINGS:** 2
CALORIES: 120 | CARBS: 7 G | FAT: 7 G | PROTEIN: 6 G | FIBER: 1 G

- 1 large zucchini, sliced into rounds
- ¼ cup (60 ml) tomato sauce
- ½ tsp dried oregano
- ¼ tsp chili flakes
- ¼ cup (30 g) shredded mozzarella (or dairy-free alternative)
- 1 tbsp fresh basil, chopped
- 1 tbsp parmesan
- ½ tsp garlic powder

1. Preheat oven to 200°C (400°F). Arrange zucchini slices on a baking tray.
2. Spread tomato sauce on each slice. Top with mozzarella, oregano, garlic powder, chili flakes, basil, and parmesan.
3. Bake for 8–10 minutes, or until cheese melts and bubbles. Serve hot.

TROPICAL BERRY BLISS YOGURT BOWL

GF, VG, DF, V

PREP TIME: 5 mins **COOK TIME:** 0 min **SERVINGS:** 4

CALORIES: 280 KCAL | PROTEIN: 6G | CARBS: 40G | FAT: 9G | FIBER: 6G

- 1 cup dairy-free yogurt (coconut or almond yogurt)
- 1 banana, sliced into thin rounds
- ½ cup strawberries, sliced
- ¼ cup raspberries
- ¼ cup mango cubes
- 1 tbsp chia seeds
- 1 tbsp pumpkin seeds
- 1 tbsp sunflower seeds
- 1 tbsp honey or maple syrup
- 1 tbsp granola (gluten-free if necessary)
- Pinch of cinnamon
- ¼ cup chopped almonds or walnuts

1. Divide the dairy-free yogurt into two bowls. Place banana slices, strawberries, raspberries, and mango cubes on top of the yogurt.
2. Sprinkle chia seeds, pumpkin seeds, sunflower seeds, and granola over the fruits. Drizzle with honey or maple syrup and lightly dust with cinnamon. Sprinkle with chopped nuts if desired.

MATCHA COCONUT BLISS BALLS

VG, GF, DF, SF, V

PREP TIME: 15 mins **COOK TIME:** 0 min

SERVINGS: 12 balls

CALORIES: 80 | CARBS: 4 G | FAT: 7 G | PROTEIN: 2 G | FIBER: 1 G

- 1 cup (100 g) shredded coconut
- ¼ cup (30 g) almond flour
- ¼ cup (60 ml) coconut cream
- 1 tsp matcha powder
- 1 tbsp maple syrup
- ½ tsp vanilla extract
- 1 tbsp hemp seeds
- Pinch of sea salt

1. Mix shredded coconut, almond flour, coconut cream, matcha powder, maple syrup, vanilla extract, hemp seeds, and a pinch of sea salt in a bowl to form a sticky dough.
2. Roll the dough into 12 small balls. Coat with extra shredded coconut.
3. Chill in the refrigerator for at least 15 minutes before serving.

CRISPY SUSHI ROLLS

VG, DF, V

PREP TIME: 5 mins **COOK TIME:** 5 mins **SERVINGS:** 4

CALORIES: 330 KCAL | PROTEIN: 8G | CARBS: 45G | FAT: 10G | FIBER: 4G

- 1 cup sushi rice
- 1 ¼ cups water
- 1 tbsp rice vinegar
- 1 tsp sugar
- ½ tsp salt
- 4 nori sheets
- 1 cucumber, julienned
- 1 avocado, sliced
- ½ cup shrimp or tofu (optional)
- 1 cup panko breadcrumbs
- ¼ cup cornstarch
- 1 tbsp flour
- ½ tsp salt
- ¼ tsp pepper
- 1-2 tbsp vegetable oil
- ½ cup water
- 1 tbsp sesame seeds
- 1-2 tbsp soy sauce
- 1-2 tbsp pickled ginger
- 1 tsp wasabi

4. Rinse rice, cook with water, then mix in vinegar, sugar, and salt, and let cool.
5. Lay nori, spread rice, add cucumber, avocado, and protein. Roll tightly.
6. Mix panko, cornstarch, flour, salt, and pepper. Dip rolls in water, coat in mixture.
7. Heat oil, fry rolls for 2-3 minutes per side until golden.
8. Slice rolls and serve with soy sauce, ginger, and wasabi.

TURMERIC HUMMUS WITH VEGGIE STICKS

GF, VG, DF, V

PREP TIME: 10 mins **COOK TIME:** 0 min **SERVINGS:** 4

CALORIES: 180 KCAL | PROTEIN: 6G | CARBS: 20G | FAT: 8G | FIBER: 5G

- 1 can of chickpeas (drained and rinsed)
- 1 tbsp tahini
- 1 tbsp olive oil
- 1 clove garlic
- 1 tsp ground turmeric
- Juice of 1 lemon
- Carrot, cucumber, and bell pepper sticks
- Salt and pepper to taste

1. Blend the chickpeas, tahini, garlic, turmeric, lemon juice, and olive oil until smooth.
2. Add a little water to adjust the consistency. Season with salt and pepper to taste.
3. Serve with fresh veggie sticks for dipping.

AVOCADO AND BERRY SMOOTHIE

GF, NF

PREP TIME: 5 mins **COOK TIME:** 0 min **SERVINGS:** 2

CALORIES: 220 KCAL | PROTEIN: 4G | CARBS: 20G | FAT: 16G | FIBER: 10G

- 1 ripe avocado
- 1 cup frozen mixed berries
- 1 cup almond milk (or any plant-based milk)
- 1 tbsp chia seeds
- 1 tsp honey
- Optional: ½ tsp cinnamon
- Handful of spinach

1. Blend all until smooth.
2. Pour into glasses and enjoy chilled.

GOLDEN MILK LATTE

GF, NF

PREP TIME: 5 mins **COOK TIME:** 5 mins **SERVINGS:** 2

CALORIES: 80 KCAL | PROTEIN: 1G | CARBS: 10G | FAT: 4G | FIBER: 1G

- 2 cups unsweetened almond milk
- 1 tsp ground turmeric
- ½ tsp ground ginger
- ½ tsp cinnamon
- 1 tsp honey
- Pinch of black pepper

1. Heat almond milk in a saucepan over low heat.
2. Whisk in turmeric, ginger, cinnamon, and black pepper.
3. Sweeten with honey if desired, and serve warm.

BLUEBERRY ALMOND BUTTER CAKE

GF, DF

PREP TIME: 5 mins **COOK TIME:** 25 mins **SERVINGS:** 6

CALORIES: 250 KCAL | PROTEIN: 6G | CARBS: 30G | FAT: 10G | FIBER: 4G

- 200g blueberries
- 100g almond butter
- 150g all-purpose flour (or almond flour for gluten-free)
- 1 tsp baking powder
- 100ml almond milk (or regular milk)
- 2 eggs
- 50g honey or maple syrup
- 1 tsp vanilla extract

1. Preheat the oven to 180°C (350°F) and grease a 9-inch pie dish or round pan.
2. In a bowl, whisk together almond butter, eggs, honey, vanilla, and almond milk until smooth.
3. Add flour and baking powder, mixing until just combined. Fold in the blueberries gently.
4. Pour the batter into the prepared dish and smooth the top.
5. Bake for 20-25 minutes, or until a toothpick inserted into the center comes out clean.
6. Cool slightly before slicing and serving.

SWEET PEPPER GUACAMOLE CUPS

VG, GF, DF, SF, V

PREP TIME: 10 mins **COOK TIME:** 0 min **SERVINGS:** 2

CALORIES: 140 | CARBS: 10 G | FAT: 12 G | PROTEIN: 3 G | FIBER: 5 G

- 3 mini sweet peppers, halved and deseeded
- 1 ripe avocado
- 1 tbsp lime juice
- 1 tsp garlic powder
- 1 tbsp chopped cilantro
- Salt to taste
- ¼ tsp smoked paprika
- 1 tbsp red onion, finely diced
- 1 tbsp pomegranate seeds

1. Mash avocado with lime juice, garlic powder, smoked paprika, cilantro, and salt.
2. Stir in diced red onion and pomegranate seeds.
3. Spoon the guacamole into sweet pepper halves. Serve immediately.

SPICED SWEET POTATO AND LENTIL CAKES

VG, GF, DF, SF, NF, V

PREP TIME: 20 mins **COOK TIME:** 15 mins **SERVINGS:** 4

CALORIES: 210 | CARBS: 30 G | FAT: 7 G | PROTEIN: 8 G | FIBER: 7 G

- 1 cup (200 g) cooked red lentils
- 1 cup (200 g) mashed sweet potato
- ¼ cup (30 g) chickpea flour
- 1 clove garlic, minced
- ½ tsp smoked paprika
- ¼ tsp turmeric powder
- 2 tbsp chopped parsley
- ¼ tsp ground cumin
- 1 tbsp olive oil for frying
- Salt and black pepper, to taste
- ¼ cup (40 g) cooked quinoa
- 1 tbsp nutritional yeast

1. Combine lentils, sweet potato, chickpea flour, quinoa, garlic, spices, parsley, and nutritional yeast in a bowl to make a thick batter. Add more flour if needed.
2. Heat olive oil in a skillet over medium heat. Shape the mixture into small patties.
3. Fry each patty for 3–4 minutes per side until golden. Serve with dairy-free yogurt or chutney.

ANTI-INFLAMMATORY GREEN SMOOTHIE

GF, DF, VG, V

PREP TIME: 5 mins **COOK TIME:** 0 min **SERVINGS:** 2

CALORIES: 180 KCAL | PROTEIN: 4G | CARBS: 20G | FAT: 10G | FIBER: 7G

- 1 cup spinach
- ½ avocado
- ½ cucumber
- ¼ cup frozen pineapple or mango chunks
- 1 tbsp chia seeds
- 1 cup unsweetened almond milk
- 1 tsp fresh ginger (grated)
- Optional: A drizzle of honey or a squeeze of lemon for extra zest

1. Add all to a blender.
2. Blend until smooth, adding more almond milk if needed for desired consistency.
3. Serve cold and enjoy!

MANGO CHIA PUDDING

VG, GF, DF, SF, V (OPTIONAL)

PREP TIME: 5 mins (plus chilling)
COOK TIME: 0 min **SERVINGS:** 2

CALORIES: 160 | CARBS: 18 G | FAT: 6 G | PROTEIN: 4 G | FIBER: 5 G

- 1 cup (240 ml) almond milk
- 3 tbsp chia seeds
- ½ cup (100 g) fresh mango purée
- 1 tsp honey or maple syrup
- ¼ tsp ground cinnamon
- ¼ tsp vanilla extract
- 1 tbsp shredded coconut (for topping)

1. Mix almond milk, chia seeds, honey, cinnamon, and vanilla in a bowl. Stir well and let it rest for 10 minutes, stirring occasionally.
2. Pour the mixture into serving glasses and top with mango purée. Refrigerate for at least 15 minutes. Serve chilled with shredded coconut on top.

TAHINI BANANA RICE CAKES

VG, GF, DF, SF, V (OPTIONAL)

PREP TIME: 5 mins **COOK TIME:** 0 min **SERVINGS:** 2

CALORIES: 180 | CARBS: 21 G | FAT: 10 G | PROTEIN: 4 G | FIBER: 4 G

- 2 rice cakes
- 2 tbsp tahini
- 1 small banana, sliced
- 1 tsp chia seeds
- 1 tbsp almond butter
- ½ tsp cinnamon
- 1 tbsp honey or maple syrup

1. Spread tahini and almond butter (if using) on each rice cake.
2. Top with banana slices, sprinkle with chia seeds, cinnamon, and drizzle with honey or maple syrup. Serve immediately.

Scan this QR code to download recipes with vibrant, full-color photos, '**A Handbook of 100 Classic Anti-Inflammatory Recipes with Full Colored Pictures**'

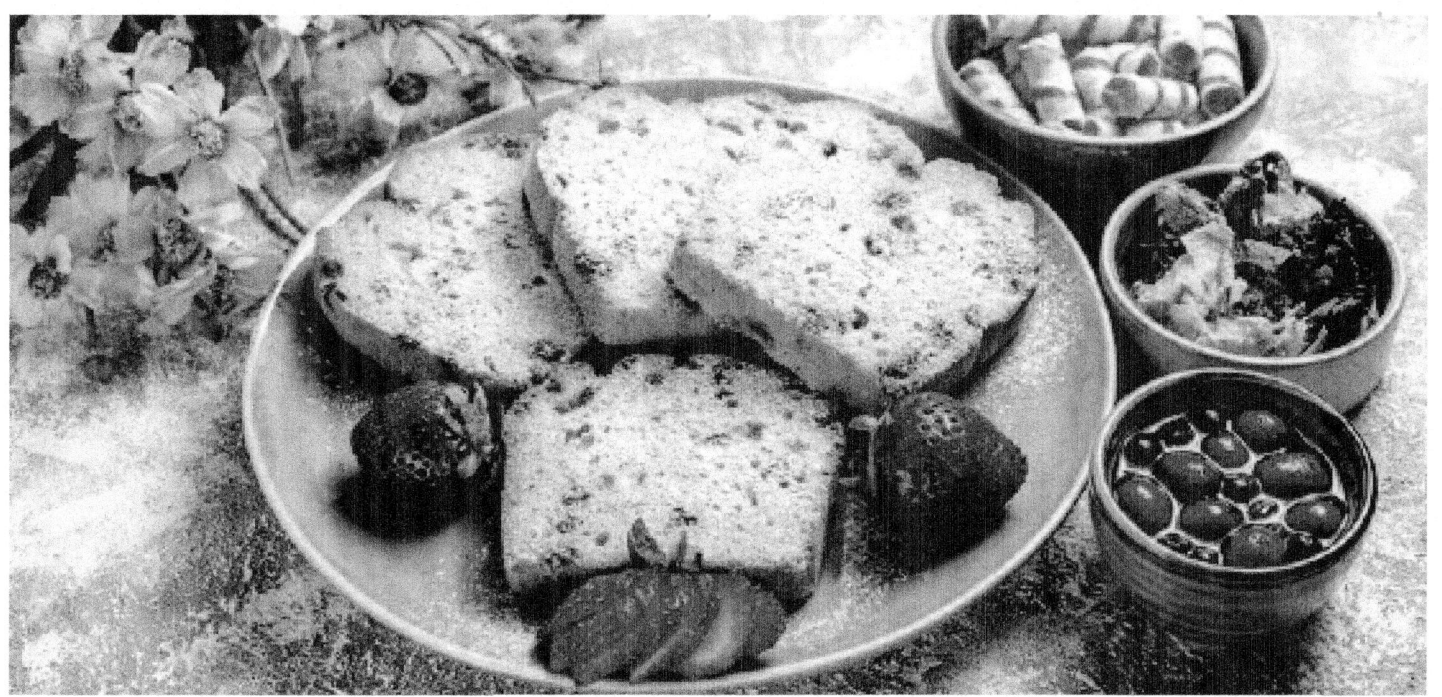

CHAPTER 14

DESSERTS

"Glorious days beckon... Indulge in sweetness that heals, not harms."

Desserts are delicious treats made with ingredients known to reduce inflammation and support overall health. These recipes typically incorporate natural sweeteners, antioxidant-rich fruits, healthy fats, and whole grains.

They aim to satisfy your sweet tooth without spiking blood sugar or causing inflammation, which is often triggered by refined sugars, processed flours, or unhealthy fats.

TIPS

- **SUBSTITUTE:** Swap refined sugar with natural options like honey, maple syrup, or dates. They offer sweetness while providing antioxidants and other health benefits.

- **STORAGE:** Many anti-inflammatory desserts, especially those made with fresh fruit, nut butters, or healthy fats, are best stored in an airtight container in the refrigerator. This helps maintain freshness and prevent spoilage. Desserts like chia pudding, avocado chocolate mousse, or berry parfaits last about 3-5 days in the fridge.

SPICED BAKED PEARS WITH WALNUTS

GF, DF, VG (IF OMITTED HONEY), V

PREP TIME: 5 mins **COOK TIME:** 20 mins **SERVINGS:** 4

CALORIES: 150 KCAL | PROTEIN: 3G | CARBS: 20G | FAT: 9G | FIBER: 5G

- 2 ripe pears, halved and cored
- ¼ cup walnuts, chopped
- 1 tbsp maple syrup
- ½ tsp ground cinnamon
- ¼ tsp ground nutmeg
- ½ tsp fresh lemon zest
- 1 tbsp coconut oil, melted
- Optional: Coconut yogurt for serving
- Optional garnish: Drizzle honey and a sprinkle of crushed pistachios for added crunch and berries if desired

1. Preheat the oven to 350°F (175°C).
2. Arrange the pear halves in a baking dish.
3. In a small bowl, mix the walnuts, maple syrup, cinnamon, nutmeg, lemon zest, and melted coconut oil.
4. Spoon the walnut mixture into the center of each pear half.
5. Bake for 20 minutes until the pears are tender and golden.
6. Serve warm, optionally with a dollop of coconut yogurt, a drizzle of honey, and a sprinkle of crushed pistachios and berries for an extra layer of flavor.

CINNAMON SWEET POTATO BROWNIES

GF, DF, V

PREP TIME: 5 mins **COOK TIME:** 25 mins **SERVINGS:** 9

CALORIES: 150 KCAL | PROTEIN: 4G | CARBS: 20G | FAT: 7G | FIBER: 3G

- 1 cup cooked sweet potato (mashed)
- ¼ cup almond butter
- ¼ cup cocoa powder
- ¼ cup maple syrup
- 1 tsp ground cinnamon
- ½ tsp ground nutmeg
- 1 tsp vanilla extract
- ½ tsp baking powder
- Optional: Dark chocolate chips and a sprinkle of sea salt

1. Preheat your oven to 350°F (175°C) and lightly grease a small baking dish.
2. In a mixing bowl, combine the mashed sweet potato, almond butter, cocoa powder, maple syrup, cinnamon, nutmeg, vanilla extract, and baking powder. Mix until smooth.
3. Stir in dark chocolate chips if using, and pour the batter into the prepared baking dish, spreading it evenly.
4. Bake for 20-25 minutes, or until a toothpick inserted into the center comes out clean.
5. Let cool before cutting into squares for the perfect texture.

STRAWBERRY COCONUT ICE CREAM

VG, GF, DF, SF, NF, V

PREP TIME: 10 mins **COOK TIME:** 0 min

FREEZING TIME: 30 mins **SERVINGS:** 2

CALORIES: 140 | CARBS: 22 G | FAT: 8 G | PROTEIN: 2 G | FIBER: 6 G

- 2 cups frozen strawberries
- ½ cup coconut cream
- ¼ cup maple syrup
- ½ tsp vanilla extract

1. Blend frozen strawberries, coconut cream, maple syrup, and vanilla extract in a food processor until smooth and creamy.
2. Spoon into a container and freeze for 30 minutes for a firmer texture.
3. Serve immediately for a soft-serve consistency or freeze longer for a harder texture.

TURMERIC COCONUT ENERGY BALLS

GF (IF USING GF OATS), DF, VG (IF OMITTED HONEY), V

PREP TIME: 15 mins **COOK TIME:** 0 min **SERVINGS:** 10

CALORIES: 180 KCAL | PROTEIN: 5G | CARBS: 16G FAT: 11G | FIBER: 4G

- 1 cup rolled oats (use gluten-free if needed)
- ½ cup almond butter
- ¼ cup unsweetened shredded coconut
- 2 tbsp honey or maple syrup (for vegan)
- 1 tsp ground turmeric
- 1 tsp ground cinnamon
- 1 tbsp chia seeds
- 2 tbsp coconut oil
- Optional: ¼ cup dark chocolate chips for added richness

1. Mix all the in a bowl until well combined.
2. Roll the mixture into small balls (about 1 inch in diameter).
3. Chill in the refrigerator for 15 minutes before serving.

NO-BAKE LEMON CHEESECAKE

VG, GF, DF, SF, V

PREP TIME: 15 mins **COOK TIME:** 0 min
CHILL TIME: 30 mins **SERVINGS:** 6
CALORIES: 220 | CARBS: 18 G | FAT: 18 G | PROTEIN: 4 G | FIBER: 5 G

For the crust:
- ½ cup shredded coconut
- ¼ cup almond flour
- 2 tbsp coconut flour
- ¼ cup coconut oil, melted

For the filling:
- 1 ½ cups cashews, soaked for 2 hours
- ¼ cup coconut oil, melted
- ¼ cup maple syrup
- ¼ cup lemon juice
- 1 tsp lemon zest

1. In a bowl, mix the shredded coconut, almond flour, and coconut flour. Add melted coconut oil and stir until the mixture holds together when pressed.
2. Press the crust mixture firmly into the bottom of serving dishes or a pie dish. Refrigerate while preparing the filling.
3. Drain the soaked cashews and blend them with melted coconut oil, maple syrup, lemon juice, and lemon zest until smooth and creamy.
4. Pour the cheesecake filling over the chilled crust and spread it evenly.
5. Refrigerate for at least 30 minutes to allow the cheesecake to set before serving.

MANGO BANANA SMOOTHIE BOWL

GF (IF USING CERTIFIED GF), DF, VG (IF OMITTED HONEY), V

PREP TIME: 10 mins **COOK TIME:** 0 min **SERVINGS:** 1
CALORIES: 230 KCAL | PROTEIN: 5G | CARBS: 38G | FAT: 10G | FIBER: 8G

- 1 frozen banana
- ½ cup mango chunks (frozen or fresh)
- ½ tsp ground turmeric
- ½ tsp freshly grated ginger (or ground ginger)
- ½ cup coconut milk
- 1 tbsp chia seeds
- 1 tbsp shredded coconut
- ¼ tsp cinnamon
- 1 tbsp almond butter
- Toppings: Fresh berries, granola, sliced almonds, a drizzle of honey or maple syrup

1. Blend the frozen banana, mango, turmeric, ginger, coconut milk, cinnamon, and almond butter until smooth and creamy.
2. Pour the smoothie into a bowl and sprinkle chia seeds, shredded coconut, and your favorite toppings like fresh berries, granola, or sliced almonds.
3. Enjoy immediately and savor the refreshing flavors!

APPLE CINNAMON COOKIES

VG, GF, DF, SF, V

PREP TIME: 10 mins **COOK TIME:** 15 mins **SERVINGS:** 12
CALORIES: 120 | CARBS: 15 G | FAT: 8 G | PROTEIN: 2 G | FIBER: 4 G

- 1 cup almond flour
- ¼ cup coconut flour
- ¼ cup coconut oil, melted
- ¼ cup maple syrup
- ½ apple, grated
- 1 tsp ground cinnamon
- ¼ tsp nutmeg
- ¼ tsp vanilla extract

1. Preheat the oven to 175°C (350°F) and line a baking sheet with parchment paper.
2. Mix almond flour, coconut flour, cinnamon, nutmeg, and grated apple in a bowl.
3. Stir in melted coconut oil, maple syrup, and vanilla.
4. Drop spoonfuls of dough onto the baking sheet and flatten slightly.
5. Bake for 12–15 minutes, until golden. Let cool before serving.

BLUEBERRY CASHEW CHEESECAKE BITES

GF, DF, VG (IF OMITTED HONEY), V

PREP TIME: 15 mins **FREEZE TIME:** 2 hours **SERVINGS:** 8

CALORIES: 180 KCAL | PROTEIN: 4G | CARBS: 15G | FAT: 12G | FIBER: 3G

- ½ cup almonds
- ½ cup dates
- 1 tbsp coconut oil
- 1 cup raw cashews (soaked for at least 2 hours)
- ½ cup coconut cream
- ¼ cup maple syrup
- 1 tsp vanilla extract
- Zest of 1 lemon
- ½ cup fresh or frozen blueberries

1. Blend the almonds, dates, and coconut oil in a food processor until sticky. Press the mixture into a lined muffin tin or silicone mold to form the crust.
2. In a blender, combine the soaked cashews, coconut cream, maple syrup, vanilla extract, and lemon zest. Blend until smooth and creamy.
3. Pour the cashew mixture over the crust and top with blueberries for a burst of flavor.
4. Freeze for at least 2 hours. Let sit at room temperature for 10 minutes before serving to soften slightly.

RASPBERRY MACAROONS

VG, GF, DF, SF, V

PREP TIME: 10 mins **COOK TIME:** 15 mins **SERVINGS:** 12

CALORIES: 150 | CARBS: 13 G | FAT: 11 G | PROTEIN: 2 G | FIBER: 3 G

- 2 cups shredded coconut
- ¼ cup maple syrup
- ¼ cup almond flour
- ½ tsp vanilla extract
- ¼ cup raspberries, crushed
- 1 tbsp coconut oil

1. Preheat the oven to 180°C (350°F) and line a baking tray with parchment paper.
2. Mix shredded coconut, maple syrup, almond flour, vanilla, and coconut oil in a bowl.
3. Gently fold in crushed raspberries.
4. Form small mounds with your hands and place them on the baking tray.
5. Bake for 12–15 minutes until golden. Let cool before serving.

CHOCOLATE COVERED STRAWBERRIES WITH MATCHA

VG, GF, DF, SF, V

PREP TIME: 10 mins **COOK TIME:** 0 min
CHILL TIME: 20 mins **SERVINGS:** 8

CALORIES: 120 | CARBS: 15 G | FAT: 9 G | PROTEIN: 2 G | FIBER: 3 G

- 1 cup dark chocolate (70% or more)
- 1 tbsp coconut oil
- ½ tsp matcha powder
- 8 medium strawberries
- ¼ cup chopped pistachios
- 1 tbsp shredded coconut

1. Melt dark chocolate and coconut oil in a heatproof bowl over simmering water (double boiler method).
2. Stir in matcha powder until fully combined.
3. Dip each strawberry into the melted chocolate, coating halfway.
4. Optional: Roll the coated strawberries in chopped pistachios or shredded coconut.
5. Place on parchment paper and refrigerate for 20 minutes to set.

CHOCOLATE BANANA MUFFINS

VG, GF, DF, SF, V

PREP TIME: 10 mins **COOK TIME:** 20 mins **SERVINGS:** 8

CALORIES: 160 | CARBS: 24 G | FAT: 8 G | PROTEIN: 4 G | FIBER: 5 G

- 2 ripe bananas, mashed
- ½ cup almond flour
- ¼ cup coconut flour
- ¼ cup cocoa powder
- ¼ cup maple syrup
- ¼ cup almond milk
- ½ tsp vanilla extract
- 1 tsp baking powder
- ¼ cup dark chocolate chips

1. Preheat the oven to 180°C (350°F) and line a muffin tin with paper liners.
2. In a bowl, mix mashed bananas, almond flour, coconut flour, cocoa powder, maple syrup, almond milk, vanilla extract, and baking powder.
3. Fold in chocolate chips and spoon the batter into the muffin tin.
4. Bake for 18–20 minutes until a toothpick comes out clean.

AVOCADO CHOCOLATE MOUSSE

GF, DF, VG (IF OMITTED HONEY), V

PREP TIME: 2 mins **COOK TIME:** 0 min **SERVINGS:** 2
CALORIES: 220 KCAL | PROTEIN: 4G | CARBS: 20G | FAT: 16G | FIBER: 10G

- 2 ripe avocados
- ¼ cup unsweetened cocoa powder
- 3 tbsp maple syrup
- 1 tsp vanilla extract
- Pinch of sea salt
- Optional: Fresh berries or crushed nuts for topping

1. Blend all in a food processor until smooth.
2. Taste and adjust sweetness if needed.
3. Chill for 15 minutes in the fridge before serving.

COCONUT POPSICLES

GF, DF, NF, VG (IF OMITTED HONEY), V

PREP TIME: 5 mins **FREEZE TIME:** 3 hours **SERVINGS:** 4
CALORIES: 100 KCAL | PROTEIN: 1G | CARBS: 5G | FAT: 9G | FIBER: 1G

- 1 ½ cups coconut milk
- 1 tbsp ground turmeric
- ½ tsp ground cinnamon
- 1 tbsp maple syrup or honey
- 1 tsp vanilla extract

1. Blend all until smooth.
2. Pour the mixture into popsicle molds and freeze for at least 3 hours.
3. Enjoy directly from the freezer.

DARK CHOCOLATE ALMOND BARK

GF, VG, V, DF, SF

PREP TIME: 5 mins **CHILL TIME:** 15 mins **SERVINGS:** 6
CALORIES: 160 KCAL | PROTEIN: 4G | CARBS: 14G | FAT: 11G | FIBER: 5G

- 1 cup dark chocolate (70% or higher, chopped)
- ½ cup almonds (roughly chopped)
- ¼ cup dried cranberries or dried orange zest
- ¼ tsp chili flakes
- Pinch of sea salt

1. Melt the dark chocolate in a microwave or double boiler.
2. Stir in the chopped almonds, dried cranberries or orange zest, and chili flakes.
3. Spread the mixture onto parchment paper and sprinkle with sea salt.
4. Let it set in the refrigerator for 15 minutes until firm.

PUMPKIN SPICE ENERGY BITES

VG, GF, DF, SF, V

PREP TIME: 10 mins **COOK TIME:** 0 min
CHILL TIME: 20 mins **SERVINGS:** 12
CALORIES: 150 | CARBS: 20 G | FAT: 8 G | PROTEIN: 4 G | FIBER: 5 G

- 1 cup rolled oats
- ¼ cup pumpkin puree
- ¼ cup almond butter
- ¼ cup maple syrup
- ½ tsp pumpkin pie spice
- ¼ tsp vanilla extract
- ¼ cup sunflower seeds

1. Combine oats, pumpkin puree, almond butter, maple syrup, pumpkin pie spice, and vanilla in a bowl.
2. Roll the mixture into small balls and coat with sunflower seeds.
3. Refrigerate for 20 minutes to firm up.

ALMOND FUDGE BARS

VG, GF, SF, NF, V

PREP TIME: 10 mins **COOK TIME:** 10 mins
CHILL TIME: 1 hour **SERVINGS:** 8
CALORIES: 180 | CARBS: 12 G | FAT: 14 G | PROTEIN: 4 G | FIBER: 5 G

- 1/2 cup coconut flour
- 1/4 cup almond butter
- 1/4 cup maple syrup
- 1/4 cup shredded coconut
- 1/4 cup dark chocolate chips
- 1/2 tsp vanilla extract
- 1/8 tsp sea salt

1. In a medium bowl, mix almond butter, maple syrup, coconut flour, shredded coconut, vanilla, and sea salt.
2. Stir until a dough forms.
3. Press the dough into a lined baking dish, smoothing the top.
4. Melt chocolate chips and drizzle on top, if desired.
5. Refrigerate for at least 1 hour until firm. Slice into bars and serve.

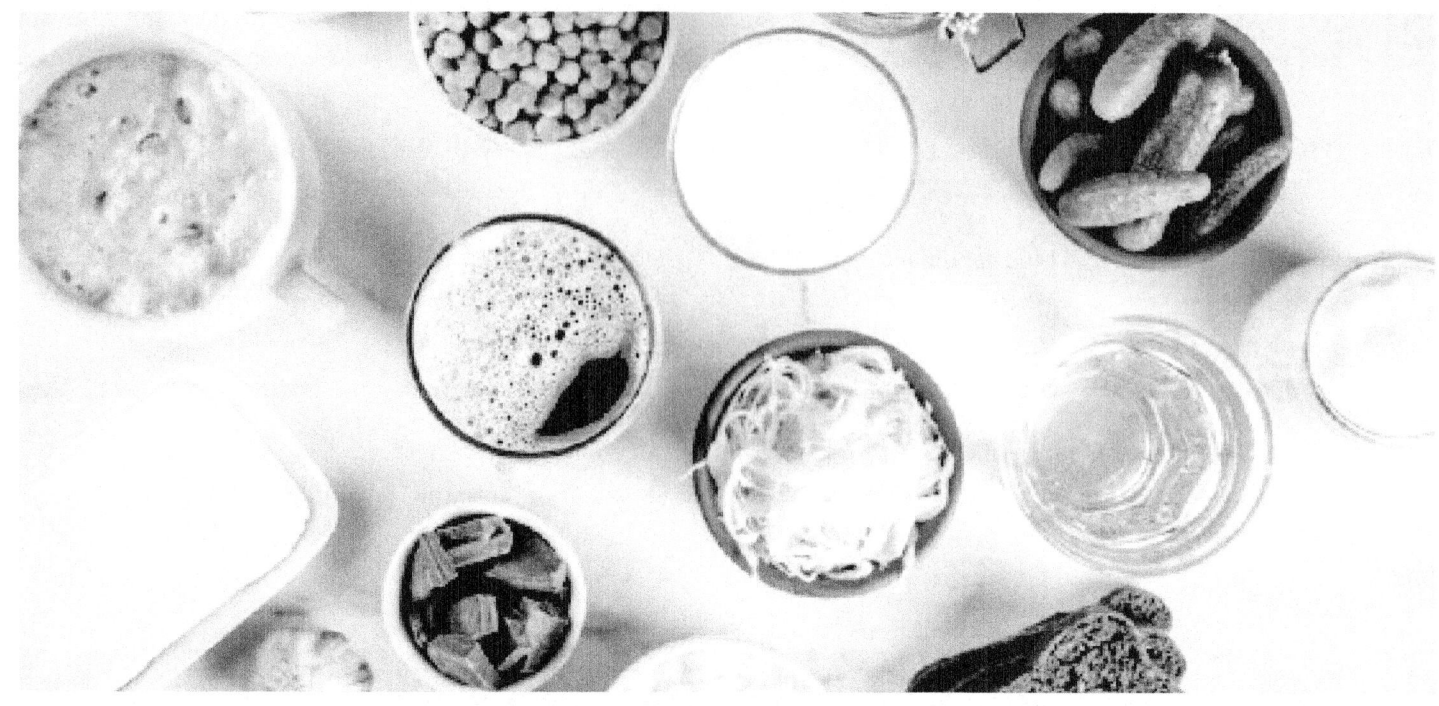

CHAPTER 15

FERMENTED FOODS

"Let the magic of fermentation transform your plate—where each bite brings harmony, health, and natural sweetness."

Fermented foods are a great addition to an anti-inflammatory diet, supporting gut health and boosting immunity. Rich in probiotics, they promote a balanced microbiome, helping reduce inflammation.

Ingredients like kimchi, sauerkraut, kefir, and kombucha nourish the digestive system, reduce bloating, and support wellness.

These foods offer both savory and subtly sweet flavors, enhancing meals while keeping inflammation in check.

TIPS:

- **HEALTHY OPTIONS:** Fermented foods like kefir, kimchi, sauerkraut, kombucha, tempeh, miso, and pickled vegetables are rich in probiotics that support gut health and reduce inflammation. For healthier choices, opt for low-sugar or unsweetened varieties and select products with minimal additives.

- **STORAGE:** Store fermented foods in glass containers with tight-fitting lids in the fridge. Leave space at the top for expansion and ensure the food is submerged in brine. After fermentation, most foods last 3 to 4 weeks, with some like kimchi and sauerkraut lasting up to 2–3 months. Always check for spoilage signs like off smells or mold.

MIXED VEGETABLE PICKLES

GF, VG, DF, V

PREP TIME: 20 mins **FERMENTATION TIME:** 5-7 days **SERVINGS:** 10

CALORIES: 20 KCAL | PROTEIN: 1G | CARBS: 3G | FAT: 0G | FIBER: 2G

- 1 cup carrots, sliced into thick rounds
- 1 cup cucumbers, quartered
- 1 cup green peppers or chilies, sliced
- 1 cup cabbage, cut into chunks
- 1 cup cauliflower florets
- 4-5 garlic cloves, peeled
- 4 cups water
- ¼ cup white vinegar
- 2 tbsp salt (non-iodized, like sea salt)
- 1 tsp sugar
- 1 tsp whole black peppercorns
- 1 tsp mustard seeds

1. In a pot, heat water, salt, and sugar (if using) until dissolved. Remove from heat and let cool. Stir in vinegar.
2. In a sterilized glass jar, layer the vegetables, garlic, and spices tightly.
3. Pour the cooled brine over the vegetables, ensuring they are fully submerged. Place a small weight (like a clean stone or a smaller lid) to keep them under the liquid.
4. Seal the jar loosely and place it in a cool, dark place. Allow fermentation for 5-7 days. Check daily for bubbles or pressure buildup, releasing air if necessary.
5. After 5 days, taste the pickles. If they're tangy enough, refrigerate to slow fermentation and serve.

LABNEH WITH PITA BREAD

GF, SF, NF

PREP TIME: 10 mins **COOK TIME:** 0 min **SERVINGS:** 4

CALORIES: 180 KCAL | PROTEIN: 7G | CARBS: 12G | FAT: 12G | FIBER: 4G

- 2 cups plain full-fat yogurt (or use pre-made labneh)
- ½ tsp salt
- Olive oil for drizzling
- 1/3 cup black olives, finely chopped
- 1/3 cup green olives, finely chopped
- 1 tsp dried za'atar
- 1 tbsp fresh parsley, chopped
- 4 pita bread rounds (or gluten-free bread for a GF option)

1. If making labneh from yogurt, place yogurt in a cheesecloth-lined strainer over a bowl. Sprinkle with salt, fold the cloth over, and let it drain for 12-24 hours in the fridge until thickened. Skip this step if using pre-made labneh.
2. Spread the labneh in a shallow serving bowl, smoothing it out with the back of a spoon.
3. In a small bowl, mix black and green olives, za'atar (if using), and parsley. Spoon this mixture over the labneh.
4. Drizzle a generous amount of olive oil over the labneh and olives.
5. Serve with warm pita bread on the side for dipping. Enjoy as a snack or appetizer.

TROPICAL PINEAPPLE KOMBUCHA

GF, DF, V, NF, VG

PREP TIME: 10 mins
FERMENTATION TIME: 3-5 days **SERVINGS:** 4

CALORIES: 50 KCAL | PROTEIN: 0G | CARBS: 12G | FAT: 0G | FIBER: 1G

- 3 cups unflavored kombucha (homemade or store-bought)
- 1 cup fresh pineapple juice
- 4 pineapple chunks
- 1 tbsp fresh lime juice
- 1 tsp grated ginger
- Fresh mint leaves

1. In a mixing jar, combine pineapple juice, lime juice, and grated ginger. Mix well.
2. Pour the mixture into sterilized glass bottles, filling each about two-thirds full.
3. Top with kombucha, leaving about an inch of space at the top to allow for carbonation during fermentation.
4. Seal the bottles tightly and let them ferment at room temperature for 3-5 days. Check daily for carbonation by gently opening the bottle to release gas.
5. Once fizzy, refrigerate the kombucha to stop fermentation.
6. Serve chilled, garnished with pineapple chunks and fresh mint leaves.

QUICK STUFFED ARTICHOKES WITH RICE

GF, DF, NF, VG, V

PREP TIME: 10 mins **COOK TIME:** 20 mins **SERVINGS:** 4
CALORIES: 210 KCAL | PROTEIN: 5G | CARBS: 30G | FAT: 7G | FIBER: 5G

- 4 medium artichokes (trimmed and hollowed)
- 1 cup (200g) pre-cooked rice or microwavable rice
- 2 tbsp olive oil
- 1 small onion, finely chopped
- 2 garlic cloves, minced
- 2 tbsp fresh dill, chopped
- 1 tbsp fresh parsley, chopped
- Juice of 1 lemon
- 1 tsp salt
- 1 tsp black pepper
- 1 tsp ground cumin
- ½ cup (120ml) vegetable broth or water

1. Trim and hollow out the artichokes, removing the tough leaves and hairy choke. Rub with lemon to prevent browning.
2. Heat 1 tbsp olive oil in a pan. Sauté the onion and garlic for 2-3 minutes until softened. Mix the cooked rice with sautéed onions, dill, parsley, salt, pepper, and cumin.
3. Stuff the artichokes with the rice mixture. Press down gently to pack the filling.
4. Place the stuffed artichokes upright in a wide pan. Add the vegetable broth, remaining olive oil, and a squeeze of lemon juice.
5. Cover the pan and simmer over medium heat for 15-20 minutes, until the artichokes are tender. Add a little more broth if needed.
6. Serve immediately with a garnish of fresh dill and lemon wedges.

GINGER-GLAZED TEMPEH

GF, VG, NF, DF, V

PREP TIME: 5 mins **CHILL TIME:** 15 mins **SERVINGS:** 6
CALORIES: 220 KCAL | PROTEIN: 14G | CARBS: 12G | FAT: 14G | FIBER: 3G

- 1 block (8 oz) tempeh, cut into cubes
- 2 tbsp coconut oil or olive oil
- 3 cloves garlic, minced
- 1-inch piece ginger, grated
- 1 red chili, thinly sliced
- 3 tbsp tamari or low-sodium soy sauce
- 2 tbsp maple syrup
- 1 tsp turmeric powder
- 1 tbsp apple cider vinegar
- ¼ cup water
- 1 green chili, thinly sliced
- 1 tsp sesame seeds

1. Heat oil in a skillet over medium heat. Add tempeh cubes and cook until golden brown on all sides (5-7 minutes). Remove and set aside.
2. In the same skillet, sauté garlic, ginger, and red chili for 1-2 minutes until fragrant.
3. Mix tamari, maple syrup, turmeric, apple cider vinegar, and water in a small bowl. Pour the mixture into the skillet.
4. Add the cooked tempeh back to the skillet. Stir to coat the tempeh evenly with the sauce. Simmer for 3-4 minutes until the sauce thickens.
5. Garnish with green chili and sesame seeds. Serve hot with steamed vegetables or rice.

FERMENTED BERRY AND LAVENDER INFUSED WATER

GF, DF, SF, NF

PREP TIME: 5 mins **COOK TIME:** 0 min
FERMENTATION TIME: 1 day **SERVINGS:** 2
CALORIES: 30 | CARBS: 7 G | FAT: 0 G | PROTEIN: 1 G | FIBER: 2 G

- 1/2 cup mixed berries (blueberries, raspberries, strawberries)
- 1 tsp dried lavender flowers
- 1 cup filtered water
- 1 tbsp apple cider vinegar
- 1/2 tsp honey

1. Combine the berries, lavender, water, apple cider vinegar, and honey in a jar.
2. Let it ferment for 24 hours at room temperature.
3. Strain and serve over ice.

MISO SOUP WITH TEMPEH AND ZUCCHINI

VG, GF, DF, V

PREP TIME: 15 mins **COOK TIME:** 0 min
FERMENTATION TIME: 1-2 days **SERVINGS:** 4

CALORIES: 200 | CARBS: 18 G | FAT: 11 G | PROTEIN: 12 G | FIBER: 5 G

- 2 cups vegetable broth
- 2 tbsp miso paste (red or white)
- 100g tempeh, cubed
- ½ cup sliced zucchini
- 1 tbsp tamari (or soy sauce for non-GF)
- ¼ cup sliced green onions
- ½ tsp garlic powder
- 1 tsp grated ginger
- 1 clove garlic, minced
- 1 tsp sesame oil

1. In a pot, bring the vegetable broth to a simmer over medium heat.
2. Add the miso paste and whisk until fully dissolved.
3. Stir in tamari, sesame oil, garlic powder, and ginger. Let it simmer for 5 minutes.
4. Add the cubed tempeh, zucchini, and garlic. Cook for another 10 minutes until vegetables are tender and tempeh is heated through.
5. Garnish with sliced green onions before serving.

TANGY SAUERKRAUT SLAW

GF, DF, VG, NF, V

PREP TIME: 10 mins **COOK TIME:** 0 min **SERVINGS:** 4

CALORIES: 100 KCAL | PROTEIN: 2G | CARBS: 10G | FAT: 7G | FIBER: 3G

- 2 cups sauerkraut (with shredded carrot)
- 1 cup shredded white cabbage
- 1 tbsp olive oil
- 1 tbsp apple cider vinegar
- ½ tsp Dijon mustard
- ¼ tsp black pepper
- ¼ tsp caraway seeds

1. In a large mixing bowl, combine sauerkraut and shredded white cabbage.
2. In a small bowl, whisk together olive oil, apple cider vinegar, Dijon mustard, and black pepper.
3. Pour the dressing over the sauerkraut mixture and toss well to coat evenly.
4. Sprinkle with caraway seeds if using. Let the slaw sit for at least 10 minutes for the flavors to blend.
5. Serve as a side dish or topping for sandwiches or bowls.

BEETROOT YOGURT SMOOTHIE

GF, NF

PREP TIME: 5 mins **COOK TIME:** 10 mins
SERVINGS: 1

CALORIES: 230 KCAL | PROTEIN: 8G | CARBS: 35G | FAT: 6G | FIBER: 5G

- 1 medium beetroot (peeled and cooked)
- 1 cup plain yogurt (or dairy-free alternative)
- ½ cup unsweetened almond milk (or any milk of choice)
- ½ frozen banana
- 1 tbsp honey (or maple syrup, optional)
- A small handful of fresh parsley

1. If not pre-cooked, boil or steam the beetroot until tender, then let it cool.
2. In a blender, add the cooked beetroot, yogurt, almond milk, frozen banana, and honey (if using).
3. Blend on high speed until creamy and vibrant in color. Add more milk if needed to adjust the consistency.
4. Pour into a glass or jar, garnish with fresh parsley for an extra touch of freshness, and enjoy!

KEFIR KIWI BOWL

GF

PREP TIME: 10 mins **CHILL TIME:** 15 mins **SERVINGS:** 4

CALORIES: 386 KCAL | PROTEIN: 15G | CARBS: 50G | FAT: 15G | FIBER: 6G

- 1 cup plain kefir (or lactose-free kefir if needed)
- 1 medium kiwi, peeled and sliced
- ½ banana, sliced
- 1 tbsp chia seeds
- 2 tbsp chopped almonds or pecans
- 2 tbsp granola
- ¼ cup diced cucumber
- 1 tsp honey or maple syrup

1. Pour kefir into a serving bowl as the base.
2. Arrange the sliced kiwi and banana on one side of the bowl.
3. Add the diced cucumber, chopped almonds or pecans, and a sprinkle of granola if desired.
4. Top with chia seeds and drizzle with honey or maple syrup for a hint of sweetness.
5. Serve immediately and enjoy this nutrient-packed, refreshing breakfast!

KIMCHI FRIED RICE WITH SEAWEED AND WHITE SESAME

GF, DF, V, VG

PREP TIME: 10 mins   **COOK TIME:** 15 mins   **SERVINGS:** 4

CALORIES: 280 KCAL | PROTEIN: 6G | CARBS: 42G | FAT: 8G | FIBER: 3G

- 2 cups cooked rice (preferably day-old for best texture)
- 1 cup kimchi, chopped
- 2 tbsp kimchi juice
- 1 tbsp sesame oil
- 1 tbsp vegetable oil (or neutral oil)
- 1 green onion, finely chopped
- 2 garlic cloves, minced
- 1 tbsp soy sauce (use tamari for gluten-free)
- 1 tsp gochujang (Korean chili paste, optional)
- 1 tsp sesame seeds, toasted
- 1 sheet roasted seaweed, crumbled

1. Heat vegetable oil in a skillet, sauté garlic and onion for 1-2 minutes.
2. Add kimchi and cook for 3-4 minutes until caramelized.
3. Stir in rice, kimchi juice, soy sauce, and gochujang; mix well.
4. Drizzle with sesame oil, cook for 2-3 minutes, and heat through.
5. Garnish with green onion, sesame seeds, and seaweed. Serve hot.

WATERMELON FERMENTED SALSA

VG, GF, DF, SF, NF, V

PREP TIME: 10 mins   **COOK TIME:** 0 min | Fermentation **TIME:** 1-2 days   **SERVINGS:** 4

CALORIES: 60 | CARBS: 14 G | FAT: 0 G | PROTEIN: 1 G | FIBER: 3 G

- 1 cup diced watermelon
- 1/2 cup diced red onion
- 1/4 cup chopped cilantro
- 1 tbsp lime juice
- 1 tsp sea salt
- 1/2 tsp cumin
- 1 tbsp apple cider vinegar

1. Combine watermelon, onion, cilantro, lime juice, cumin, and sea salt in a bowl.
2. Add apple cider vinegar and stir well.
3. Place the mixture in a jar, close tightly, and let ferment for 1–2 days at room temperature.

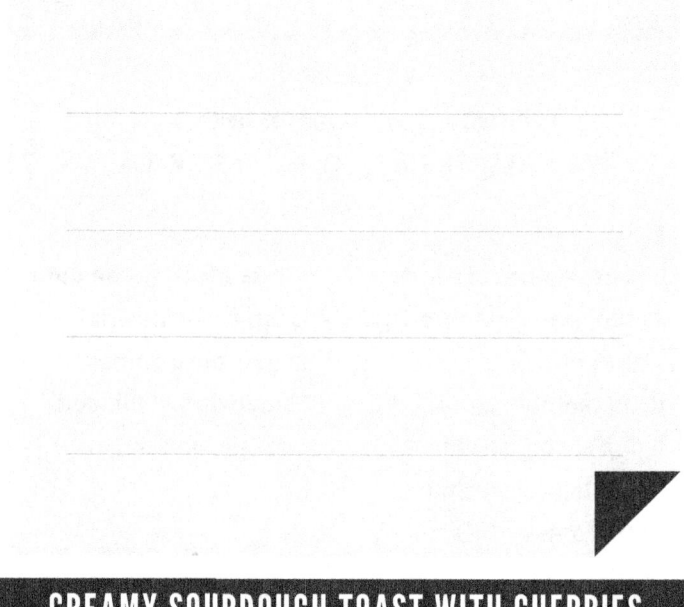

CREAMY SOURDOUGH TOAST WITH CHERRIES

GF, DF (OPTIONAL)

PREP TIME: 5 mins   **COOK TIME:** 10 mins   **SERVINGS:** 2

CALORIES: 190 KCAL | PROTEIN: 6G | CARBS: 28G | FAT: 4G | FIBER: 3G

- 4 slices of sourdough bread
- 1 tbsp olive oil or butter for toasting
- ½ cup thick yogurt (Greek or plant-based for dairy-free)
- 1 tsp honey or maple syrup
- 1 pinch salt
- 8-10 fresh cherries (pitted, whole, or halved)
- Fresh mint leaves
- ½ tsp cracked black pepper

1. Lightly brush each slice of sourdough with olive oil or butter.
2. Heat a skillet or toaster and toast the bread until golden and crispy, about 2 minutes per side.
3. In a small bowl, combine yogurt, honey (if using), and a pinch of salt. Stir until smooth and creamy.
4. Generously spread the yogurt mixture over each slice of toasted sourdough.
5. Top each toast with fresh cherries, a sprinkle of mint leaves, and cracked black pepper for a contrast of flavors.
6. Drizzle with additional honey or olive oil for extra richness. Serve immediately as a refreshing breakfast, snack, or light dessert.

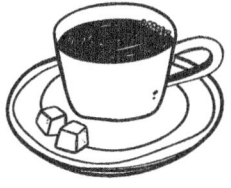

FERMENTED CARROT AND GINGER PICKLE

GF, DF, SF

PREP TIME: 15 mins **COOK TIME:** 0 min
FERMENTATION TIME: 1–2 days **SERVINGS:** 4

CALORIES: 60 | CARBS: 14 G | FAT: 1 G | PROTEIN: 1 G | FIBER: 3 G

- 2 large carrots, sliced thinly
- 1-inch fresh ginger, grated
- ¼ cup apple cider vinegar
- ¼ cup filtered water
- 1 tbsp honey
- 1 tsp salt
- ½ tsp mustard seeds
- ½ tsp turmeric

1. Place carrots and grated ginger into a jar.
2. In a bowl, combine vinegar, water, honey, salt, mustard seeds, and turmeric. Stir until the salt dissolves.
3. Pour the liquid over the carrots, ensuring they are fully submerged.
4. Close the jar and let ferment at room temperature for 1–2 days, depending on desired tanginess.

KIMCHI-INFUSED VEGGIE STIR-FRY

VG, GF, DF, V

PREP TIME: 10 mins **COOK TIME:** 10 mins
SERVINGS: 2

CALORIES: 150 | CARBS: 16 G | FAT: 9 G | PROTEIN: 4 G | FIBER: 4 G

- 1 cup kimchi, chopped
- ½ cup sliced bell pepper
- ½ cup mushrooms, sliced
- ¼ cup chopped onion
- 1 tbsp sesame oil
- 1 tbsp soy sauce
- ¼ tsp red pepper flakes
- ¼ cup sliced scallions
- 1 tbsp sesame seeds

1. Heat sesame oil in a pan over medium heat.
2. Add bell pepper, mushrooms, and onion and stir-fry for 3–4 minutes.
3. Add chopped kimchi and soy sauce, stir-fry for another 3–4 minutes.
4. Sprinkle with red pepper flakes, scallions, and sesame seeds before serving.

ANTI-INFLAMMATORY PICKLED BEETS WITH APPLE CIDER VINEGAR

GF, DF, SF

PREP TIME: 15 mins **COOK TIME:** 0 min
FERMENTATION TIME: 1–2 days **SERVINGS:** 4

CALORIES: 50 | CARBS: 12 G | FAT: 0 G | PROTEIN: 1 G | FIBER: 3 G

- 2 medium beets, peeled and sliced
- ¼ cup apple cider vinegar
- 1 tbsp honey
- ¼ tsp ground turmeric
- 1 tsp mustard seeds
- ½ cup water
- ¼ tsp sea salt

1. Place sliced beets in a jar.
2. Mix apple cider vinegar, honey, turmeric, mustard seeds, water, and salt in a bowl.
3. Pour the brine over the beets, ensuring they are fully submerged.
4. Seal the jar and leave at room temperature for 1–2 days to ferment.

ANTI-INFLAMMATORY GINGER TURMERIC KOMBUCHA SMOOTHIE

GF, DF, SF

PREP TIME: 5 mins **COOK TIME:** 0 min
SERVINGS: 2

CALORIES: 80 | CARBS: 18 G | FAT: 2 G | PROTEIN: 1 G | FIBER: 5 G

- 1 cup kombucha (ginger or turmeric flavor)
- ½ frozen banana
- ½ tsp ground turmeric
- ½ tsp grated fresh ginger
- ¼ cup almond milk
- 1 tsp chia seeds
- 1 tsp honey

1. In a blender, combine kombucha, frozen banana, turmeric, ginger, almond milk, and chia seeds.
2. Blend until smooth and creamy.
3. Taste and adjust sweetness with honey if desired. Serve immediately.

MEAL PLAN 1-7 DAYS

This 30-day meal plan is tailored for the Elimination Diet to help identify potential food sensitivities. Once you've completed the Elimination Diet, feel free to swap recipes to include 'allowed foods' that suit your preferences or dietary needs.

Day	Breakfast	Snack	Lunch	Snack	Dinner	Calories
1	Avocado Toast with Turmeric & Hemp Seeds **280kcal**	Avocado Chocolate Mousse **220kcal**	The Ultimate Arugula & Feta Salad **250kcal**	Kimchi Fried Rice with Seaweed and White Sesame **280kcal**	Grilled Salmon with Avocado Salsa **350kcal**	1380
2	Quick Chia Seed Pudding with Berries **250kcal**	Blueberry Almond Butter Cake **250kcal**	Ramen with Soft-Boiled Egg and Tofu **400kcal**	Walnuts and Dark Chocolate Bite **220kcal**	Spicy Grilled Mackerel + Turmeric-Tahini Dressing **418kcal**	1538
3	Oatmeal with Flaxseeds and Blueberries + Pineapple Smoothie with Turmeric **430kcal**	Mango Banana Smoothie Bowl **230kcal**	Chicken, Brussels Sprouts & Mushroom Salad **432kcal**	Labneh with Pita Bread **180kcal**	Lemon Garlic Baked Thyme Cod **220kcal**	1492
4	Quinoa Breakfast Bowl with Almonds and Pomegranate **320kcal**	Savory Chickpea Pancakes with Spinach **220kcal**	Mediterranean Chickpea and Cucumber Salad **230kcal**	Spicy Sweet Potato Fries **180kcal**	Pesto Baked Salmon **350kcal**	1300
5	Sweet Potato Hash with Spinach **230kcal**	Turmeric Coconut Energy Balls **180kcal**	Tuna and Egg Salad with Olives **376kcal**	Avocado and Berry Smoothie **220kcal**	Golden Grilled Chicken **280kcal**	1286
6	Quinoa Breakfast Bowl with Poached Eggs and Avocado **400kcal**	Spiced Baked Pears with Walnuts **150kcal**	Tuna Salad Lettuce Wraps **269kcal**	Cinnamon Sweet Potato Brownies **150kcal**	Paprika-Rubbed Steak **400kcal**	1369
7	Coconut Yogurt Parfait with Berries and Walnuts **220kcal**	Turmeric Hummus with Veggie Sticks **180kcal**	Spicy Tomato and Basil Soup + Shrimp Stir-fry with Vegetables **410kcal**	Dark Chocolate Almond Bark **160kcal**	Balsamic Glazed Chicken Breasts **330kcal**	1300

MEAL PLAN 8-15 DAYS

Day	Breakfast	Snack	Lunch	Snack	Dinner	Calories
8	Savory Chickpea Pancakes with Spinach **220kcal**	Anti-Inflammatory Green Smoothie **180kcal**	Cauliflower and Leek Soup + Cilantro-Lime Grilled Pork Chops **510kcal**	Coconut Popsicles **100kcal**	Seared Scallops with Garlic Spinach **350kcal**	1360
9	Egg and Buckwheat Porridge **350kcal**	Kefir Kiwi Bowl **386kcal**	Sweet Potato and Lentil Stew **220kcal**	Ginger-Glazed Tempeh **220kcal**	Cumin-Spiced Beef Tacos **350kcal**	1526
10	Oatmeal with Flaxseeds and Blueberries **250kcal**	Herb-Citrus Turkey Skewers **270kcal**	Green Detox Soup + Roasted Pumpkin with Thyme **330kcal**	Blueberry Cashew Cheesecake Bites **180kcal**	Balsamic Glazed Chicken Breasts **330kcal**	1360
11	Zucchini Quinoa Frittata **320kcal**	Avocado and Berry Smoothie **220kcal**	Butternut Squash and Chickpea Soup **250kcal**	Spiced Baked Pears with Walnuts **150kcal**	Lemon-Herb Lamb Chops **360kcal**	1300
12	Egg and Buckwheat Porridge **350kcal**	Golden Milk Latte **80kcal**	Chicken, Brussels Sprouts & Mushroom Salad **432kcal**	Blueberry Almond Butter Cake **250kcal**	Spicy Grilled Mackerel **320kcal**	1432
13	Tropical Berry Bliss Yogurt Bowl **280kcal**	Turmeric Roasted Cauliflower **110kcal**	Tuna and Egg Salad with Olives **376kcal**	Avocado Chocolate Mousse **220kcal**	Paprika-Rubbed Steak **400kcal**	1386
14	Moroccan Scrambled Eggs with Crusty Bread **300kcal**	Shrimp Stir-fry with Vegetables **230kcal**	Mediterranean Chickpea and Cucumber Salad **230kcal**	Turmeric Coconut Energy Balls **180kcal**	Spanish Chorizo and Bean Stew **320kcal**	1260
15	Quick Chia Seeds Pudding with Berries **240kcal**	Avocado Toast with Turmeric & Hemp Seeds **280kcal**	Quick Beef and Potato Stew **340kcal**	Mango Banana Smoothie Bowl **230kcal**	Pesto Baked Salmon **350kcal**	1440

MEAL PLAN 16-23 DAYS

Day	Breakfast	Snack	Lunch	Snack	Dinner	Calories
16	Stuffed Egg Wrap with Minced Pork and Vegetables **450kcal**	Mango Banana Smoothie Bowl **230kcal**	Okra and Tomato Stew **170 kcal**	Avocado Chocolate Mousse **220kcal**	Lemon-Herb Lamb Chops **360kcal**	1430
17	Coconut Yogurt Parfait with Berries and Walnuts **220kcal**	Spinach and Feta Egg Muffins **120kcal**	Kale, Avocado and Sweet Potato Bowl **220kcal**	Crispy Sushi Rolls **330kcal**	Paprika-Rubbed Steak **400kcal**	1290
18	Mediterranean Egg and Quinoa Bowl **400kcal**	Spicy Sweet Potato Fries **180kcal**	Cumin-Spiced Beef Tacos **350kcal**	Stuffed Bell Peppers with Quinoa and Black Beans **220kcal**	Seared Scallops with Garlic Spinach **350kcal**	1500
19	Avocado-Stuffed Sweet Potato Boats + Greek Yogurt **398kcal**	Avocado and Berry Smoothie **220kcal**	Sea Bass with Greek Salad **320kcal**	Herb-Citrus Turkey Skewers **270kcal**	Spicy Grilled Mackerel **320kcal**	1528
20	Avocado Toast with Turmeric & Hemp Seeds + Golden Milk Latte **340kcal**	Walnuts and Dark Chocolate Bite **220kcal**	Golden Grilled Chicken + Ginger-Soy Dressing **315kcal**	Grilled Zucchini and Eggplant with Lemon Tahini Sauce **150kcal**	Lemon Garlic Baked Thyme Cod **220kcal**	1245
21	Quick Chia Seeds Pudding with Berries **240kcal**	Blueberry Cashew Cheesecake Bites **180Kcal**	Spicy Tomato and Basil Soup+ Herb-Citrus Turkey Skewers **470kcal**	Roasted Brussels Sprouts with Balsamic Glaze **140kcal**	Cilantro-Lime Grilled Pork Chops **320kcal**	1350
22	Oatmeal with Flaxseeds and Blueberries **250kcal**	Turmeric Smoothie with Pineapple **180kcal**	Chicken, Brussels Sprouts & Mushroom Salad **420kcal**	Tuna Salad Lettuce Wraps **269kcal**	Lemon-Herb Lamb Chops **360kcal**	1479
23	Quinoa Breakfast Bowl with Almonds and Pomegranate **320kcal**	Anti-Inflammatory Green Smoothie **180kcal**	Butternut Squash and Chickpea Soup **250kcal**	Cumin-Spiced Beef Tacos **350kcal**	Grilled Salmon with Avocado Salsa **350kcal**	1450

MEAL PLAN 24-30 DAYS

Day	Breakfast	Snack	Lunch	Snacks	Dinner	Calories
24	Sweet Potato Hash with Spinach **230kcal**	Walnuts and Dark Chocolate Bite **220kcal**	Green Detox Soup+ Tangy Sauerkraut Slaw **280kcal**	Blueberry Almond Butter Cake **230kcal**	Spicy Grilled Mackerel+ Turmeric-Tahini Dressing **418kcal**	1378
25	Pineapple Smoothie with Turmeric + Avocado Toast with Turmeric & Hemp Seeds **460kcal**	Spinach and Feta Egg Muffins **120kcal**	Chicken and Vegetable Stew with Mushrooms **310kcal**	Spicy Sweet Potato Fries **180kcal**	Pesto Baked Salmon **350kcal**	1420
26	Coconut Yogurt Parfait with Berries and Walnuts **220kcal**	Avocado Chocolate Mousse **220kcal**	Mediterranean Chickpea and Cucumber Salad **230kcal**	Quick Stuffed Artichokes with Rice **210kcal**	Paprika-Rubbed Steak+ Ginger-Soy Dressing **435kcal**	1315
27	Savory Chickpea Pancakes with Spinach **220kcal**	Golden Milk Latte + Walnuts and Dark Chocolate Bite **300kcal**	Golden Grilled Chicken+ Lemon-Turmeric Vinaigrette **380kcal**	Beetroot Yogurt Smoothie **230kcal**	Seared Scallops with Garlic Spinach **350kcal**	1480
28	Quinoa Breakfast Bowl with Poached Eggs and Avocado **400kcal**	Zucchini Noodles with Pesto **200kcal**	Cilantro-Lime Grilled Pork Chops **320kcal**	Mango Banana Smoothie Bowl **230kcal**	Lemon-Herb Lamb Chops **360kcal**	1510
29	Quick Chia Seeds Pudding with Berries **240kcal**	Avocado Toast with Turmeric & Hemp Seeds **280kcal**	Egg and Millet Bowl with Spinach **330kcal**	Spiced Baked Pears with Walnuts **150kcal**	Pesto Baked Salmon **350kcal**	1350
30	Oatmeal with Flaxseeds and Blueberries + Pineapple Smoothie with Turmeric **430kcal**	Mango Banana Smoothie Bowl **230kcal**	Chicken, Brussels Sprouts & Mushroom Salad **432kcal**	Spicy Sweet Potato Fries **180kcal**	Lemon Garlic Baked Thyme Cod **220kcal**	1492

For the detailed weekly shopping lists, please go to:

https://heartbookspress.com/Anti-InflammatoryDietCookbookFreeBonuses

CONVERSIONS AND EQUIVALENTS

Precision is the secret ingredient to cooking success. Using accurate measurements not only ensures that your dishes turn out delicious every time but also keeps your anti-inflammatory meals consistent and balanced. This Cooking Conversion Chart is here to guide you through the essentials, making your time in the kitchen smooth and enjoyable.

Volume Conversions
- 1 cup = 16 tablespoons
- 1 tablespoon = 3 teaspoons
- 1 fluid ounce = 2 tablespoons = 6 teaspoons
- 1 pint = 2 cups = 16 fluid ounces
- 1 quart = 4 cups = 32 fluid ounces
- 1 gallon = 4 quarts = 16 cups = 128 fluid ounces

Weight Conversions
- 1 ounce = 28 grams
- 1 pound = 16 ounces = 454 grams
- 1 kilogram = 1000 grams = 2.2 pounds

Temperature Equivalents
Converting between temperature scales is a breeze with these simple formulas:

- To convert °F to °C: (°F - 32) × 5/9
- To convert °C to °F: (°C × 9/5) + 32

For example, 350°F converts to approximately 176.67°C. Having these conversions at your fingertips ensures your recipes turn out perfectly, no matter the temperature settings.

Common Ingredient Equivalents
Accurate ingredient measurements can make all the difference in achieving the perfect dish. Here are some useful conversions for everyday ingredients:

- 1 medium banana ≈ 1/2 cup mashed banana
- 1 large egg = 2 small eggs or 3 medium eggs
- 1 cup grated cheese = 4 ounces
- 1 cup breadcrumbs = 4 slices of bread
- 1 cup chopped nuts = 4.5 ounces
- 1 cup cooked rice = 1/2 cup uncooked rice
- 1 cup cooked pasta = 2 ounces uncooked pasta
- 1 stick of butter = 1/2 cup = 8 tablespoons = 4 ounce

CONCLUSION

As we come to the end of this journey through the world of anti-inflammatory foods, I want to thank you for allowing me to be a part of your path to better health and well-being.

This journey is more than just a collection of recipes—it's a step toward transforming your life, one nourishing meal at a time. The anti-inflammatory diet is not a restrictive plan but a celebration of flavors, colors, and the natural healing power found in wholesome ingredients.

Every dish you prepare brings you closer to a healthier, more vibrant version of yourself, and that's something to be proud of. Whether you're embracing these recipes fully or taking small, steady steps toward integrating them into your daily routine, know that every choice you make counts.

Remember that true wellness is a journey, not a destination. There will be days when it feels effortless and others when you might need a little extra encouragement. In those moments, I hope you'll return to these pages for inspiration, comfort, and a reminder of why you began this journey.

Thank you for choosing to walk this path with me. I'm grateful to have been a part of your transformation, and I hope that the meals you create from this book continue to fill your life with energy, balance, and joy.

Here's to making every bite count, to savoring the simple pleasures, and to living a life that is as rich in health as it is in flavor. To your continued journey of healing, happiness, and delicious discoveries—may you always find strength in your choices and joy in the food that sustains you.

"Let food be thy medicine, and medicine be thy food."
– Hippocrates

With gratitude and best wishes,

Elena Florenz

THANK YOU

Thank you so much for purchasing my cookbook.

You could have picked from dozens of other cookbooks but you took a chance and chose this one. I hope you've found inspiration in *The Practical Science-Backed Anti-Inflammatory Diet Cookbook for Beginners: Step by Step Plan, 200+ Super Easy Recipes & A 30-Day Meal Plan To Reset Your Cells, Immunity, and Gut Health and Ease Chronic Pain* to get you started on your journey to great health and happiness.

So THANK YOU for getting this book.

Before you go, I wanted to ask you for one small favor. Could you please consider posting a review on the platform? Posting a review is the best and easiest way to support the work of independent authors like me.

Your review will help me keep writing the kind of cookbooks that will help you get the results you want. It would mean a lot to me to hear from you.

Leave a review on
Amazon US

Leave a review on
Amazon UK

Leave a review on
Amazon CA

REFERENCES

Kasper DL, Fauci AS, Hauser SL et al. Harrison's Principles of Internal Medicine. New York: McGraw-Hill; 2015.

Pschyrembel W. Klinisches Wörterbuch. Berlin: De Gruyter; 2017.

Weil, A. (n.d.). *Anti-Inflammatory Diet & Food Pyramid*. Andrew Weil, MD

Harvard T.H. Chan School of Public Health, *Anti-Inflammatory Diet*.https://nutritionsource.hsph.harvard.edu/healthy-weight/diet-reviews/anti-inflammatory-diet/

The American Journal of Clinical Nutrition, *Mediterranean Diet's Impact on Inflammation and Disease Prevention*, Vol. 104(5), 2016.

Cleveland Clinic, *Why Omega-3 Fatty Acids Are Good for You*, 2020.

Harvard Health Publishing, *Foods That Fight Inflammation*, 2020. https://www.health.harvard.edu/staying-healthy/foods-that-fight-inflammation

Joseph, J.A., et al., *Nutrition and Brain Function: The Benefits of Antioxidants*, NIH, 2000.

Estruch, R., et al., *Mediterranean Diet and Cardiovascular Prevention: The PREDIMED Study*, AJCN, 2010.

Leeuwendaal, N.K., Stanton, C., O'Toole, P.W., & Beresford, T.P., *Fermented Foods, Health and the Gut Microbiome, Nutrients*, 2022, 14(7):1527. doi:10.3390/nu14071527. https://www.mdpi.com/2072-6643/14/7/1527

Weaver, J., *Fermented foods reduce inflammatory markers: Fermented-food diet increases microbiome diversity, decreases inflammatory proteins*, Stanford Medicine News Center, July 12, 2021. https://med.stanford.edu/news/all-news/2021/07/fermented-food-diet-increases-microbiome-diversity-lowers-inflammation

Sendl, A., *Allium Sativum (Garlic): A Natural Antibiotic and Anti-inflammatory Agent*, PubMed, 2014. Institute for Quality and Efficiency in Health Care (IQWiG); 2006-.

Furman, D., et al., *Chronic Inflammation in the Etiology of Disease Across the Life Span*, Nature Medicine, 2019.

Chen, L., et al., *Inflammation, Immunity, and the Tumor Microenvironment*, NIH, 2017.

Serhan, C.N., *Resolution of Inflammation: The Beginning Programs the End*, Nature Immunology, 2007.

Medzhitov, R., *Inflammation 2010: New Adventures of an Old Flame*, Cell, 2010.

Chen, F.M., et al., *The Role of Inflammation in the Healing and Regenerative Process*, Stem Cells International, 2016.

Serhan, C.N., et al., *Resolvins and Protectins: Omega-3 Fatty Acid-Derived Mediators in Anti-Inflammation and Cellular Regeneration*, Annual Review of Immunology, 2011.

Larsson, S.C., et al., *Dietary Factors in Inflammation and Regeneration*, NIH, 2014.

Rosenblum, M.D., *Inflammation in Autoimmune Diseases: Dysregulation and Therapeutic Targeting*, Science, 2015.

INDEX

A

Almond Butter And Ginger Dip 73
Almond Fudge Bars 85
Anti-Inflammatory Ginger Turmeric Kombucha Smoothie 91
Anti-Inflammatory Green Smoothie 79
Anti-Inflammatory Pickled Beets With Apple Cider Vinegar 91
Apple Cinnamon Cookies 83
Apple Cinnamon Quinoa Porridge 44
Asian Sesame Noodle Salad 39
Avocado And Berry Smoothie 79
Avocado And Pomegranate Salad Wrap 45
Avocado Chocolate Mousse 85
Avocado-Cilantro Sauce 75
Avocado-Stuffed Sweet Potato Boats 77
Avocado Toast With Turmeric & Hemp Seeds 44

B

Baked Grouper With Roasted Vegetables 48
Baked Herb Crusted Halibut 50
Balsamic Glazed Chicken Breasts 57
Beetroot And Blackberry Salad With Tofu And Seeds 37
Beetroot Cashew Sauce 71
Beetroot Yogurt Smoothie 89
Blackened Fish Tacos 49
Blueberry Almond Butter Cake 79
Blueberry Cashew Cheesecake Bites 84
Butternut Squash And Brussels Sprouts With Maple-Dijon Glaze 66
Butternut Squash & Chickpea Soup 30

C

Caramelized Anti-Inflammatory Vegetables 69
Carrot And Chicken Soup 28
Cauliflower And Chickpea Curry 65
Cauliflower And Leek Soup 34
Chicken And Vegetable Stew With Mushrooms 34
Chicken, Brussels Sprouts & Mushroom Salad 37
Chickpea And Tomato Stew 32
Chickpea Flour Crepes With Spiced Veggies 44
Chili Garlic Mussels In Tomato Broth 50
Chocolate Banana Muffins 84
Chocolate Covered Strawberries With Matcha 84
Cilantro-Lime Grilled Pork Chops 54
Cinnamon Sweet Potato Brownies 82
Citrus Black Bean Quinoa Salad 37
Coconut Popsicles 85
Coconut Yogurt Parfait With Berries And Walnuts 43
Creamy Bacon & Egg Spaghetti 60
Creamy Basil Avocado Sauce 71
Creamy Cashew Garlic Sauce 73
Creamy Polenta With Soft-Boiled Eggs 61
Creamy Sourdough Toast With Cherries 90
Creole Fish Stew 52
Crispy Baked Artichoke Hearts 67
Crispy Sushi Rolls 78
Crispy Sweet Potato And Black Bean Skillet 43
Crunchy Cabbage & Pumpkin Seed Slaw 36
Cumin-Spiced Beef Tacos 56
Curried Parsnip And Apple Soup 29
Curried Tofu Scramble 46

D

Dark Chocolate Almond Bark 85

E

Edamame And Seaweed Salad 40
Egg And Barley Pilaf With Dried Fruits 63
Egg And Buckwheat Porridge 62
Egg And Millet Bowl With Spinach 60
Egg And Teff Porridge With Spices And Nuts 61

F

Fermented Berry And Lavender Infused Water 88
Fermented Carrot And Ginger Pickle 90
Fluffy Omelette Rice 62

G

Garlic Butter Asparagus With Lemon Zest 67
Garlic Dill Sauce 75
Garlic Parmesan Baked Tilapia 49

Garlic Rosemary Pork Tenderloin 57
Ginger-Garlic Sautéed Spinach 68
Ginger-Glazed Tempeh 88
Ginger-Soy Dressing 74
Golden Grilled Chicken 54
Golden Milk Latte 79
Green Detox Soup 28
Green Goddess Dressing 75
Grilled Peach And Ricotta Salad 39
Grilled Salmon With Avocado Salsa 52
Grilled Zucchini And Eggplant With Lemon Tahini Sauce 68
Ground Beef Stir-Fry 55

H
Harissa Roasted Lamb Meatballs 55
Hearty Vegetable Stew 68
Herb-Citrus Turkey Skewers 54
Herb Crusted Chicken Cutlets 54
Herb-Infused Poached Eggs On Mushroom Toast 45
Homemade Tomato Ketchup 74
Honey Garlic Chicken Thighs 56
Honey Mustard Chicken Drumsticks 55

K
Kale, Avocado And Sweet Potato Bowl 38
Kefir Kiwi Bowl 89
Kimchi Fried Rice With Seaweed And White Sesame 90
Kimchi-Infused Veggie Stir-Fry 91
Korean-Style Tofu And Vegetables With Ginger Garlic Sauce 67

L
Labneh With Pita Bread 87
Lamb And Eggplant Stew 34
Lemon Garlic Baked Thyme Cod 52
Lemongrass Fish Skewers 51

Lemon-Herb Lamb Chops 57
Lemon-Turmeric Vinaigrette 74

M
Mango Banana Smoothie Bowl 83
Mango Chia Pudding 80
Matcha Coconut Bliss Balls 78
Mediterranean Chickpea And Cucumber Salad 38
Minestrone Soup 32
Minted Lentil And Cucumber Salad 40
Miso And Tofu Soup 29
Miso Glazed Eggplant And Rice Breakfast Bowl 44
Miso Soup With Tempeh And Zucchini 89
Mixed Vegetable Pickles 87
Moroccan Chicken And Apricot Stew 31
Moroccan Scrambled Eggs With Crusty Bread 63
Mushroom And Scrambled Barley Risotto 63

N
No-Bake Lemon Cheesecake 83

O
Oatmeal With Flaxseeds And Blueberries 43
Okra And Tomato Stew 30

P
Paprika-Rubbed Steak 57
Parsley Bulgur Tabbouleh 61
Pear And Walnut Salad 37
Peppercorn Crusted Steak With Garlic Butter 55
Pesto Baked Salmon 49
Pineapple Smoothie With Turmeric 45

Pomegrante Mint Sauce 72
Pumpkin And Corn Soup 30
Pumpkin Spice Energy Bites 85

Q
Quick Anti-Inflammatory Vegetable Broth With Noodles 31
Quick Beef And Potato Stew 31
Quick Broccoli Soup 29
Quick Chia Seeds Pudding With Berries 43
Quick Stuffed Artichokes With Rice 88
Quinoa Breakfast Bowl With Almonds And Pomegranate 46
Quinoa Breakfast Bowl With Poached Eggs And Avocado 59

R
Ramen With Soft-Boiled Egg And Tofu 60
Raspberry Macaroons 84
Raspberry Vinaigrette 71
Roasted Parsnips With Lime And Cilantro 69
Roasted Pumpkin With Thyme 77
Roasted Root Vegetable Medley With Herbs 66
Roasted Turnips And Carrots With Mustard 65

S
Sardines In Tomato Sauce 50
Sauteed Belgium Endives With Oranges 65
Savory Chickpea Pancakes With Spinach 45
Scrambled Egg And Farro Pilaf 59
Sea Bass With Greek Salad 51
Seared Scallops With Garlic Spinach 48
Sesame Ginger Grilled Trout 49

Sesame Ginger Sauce 72
Shakshuka With Lentils
  And Herbs 62
Shrimp Stir-Fry With Vegetables 52
Sorghum Egg Stir-Fry 61
Spanish Chorizo And Bean Stew 32
Spiced Baked Pears With
  Walnuts 82
Spiced Moroccan Ground Lamb 55
Spiced Sweet Potato And
  Lentil Cakes 80
Spicy Coconut Sauce 72
Spicy Crab Meat Stuffed Peppers 50
Spicy Crispy Calamari With
  Lime Dip 50
Spicy Egg And Couscous Bowl 61
Spicy Grilled Mackerel 48
Spicy Lemongrass Chicken Soup 33
Spicy Mango Chutney 75
Spicy Sweet Potato Fries 69
Spicy Tomato And Basil Soup 29
Spinach And Berries Salad 36
Spinach and Feta Egg Muffins 63
Stewed Vegetable With Tofu And
  Mushrooms 67
Strawberry Coconut Ice Cream 82
Stuffed Acorn Squash With Lentils
  And Pomegranate 65

Stuffed Bell Peppers With Quinoa
  And Black Beans 65
Stuffed Egg Wrap With Minced Pork
  And Vegetables 59
Sweet And Sour Turkey
  Meatballs 55
Sweet Chilli Dipping Sauce 73
Sweet Corn Egg Risotto 60
Sweet Pepper Guacamole Cups 79
Sweet Potato Hash With Spinach 45
Sweet Potato & Lentil Stew 28

T
Tahini Banana Rice Cakes 80
Tamarind Sauce 74
Tangy Sauerkraut Slaw 89
Thai Coconut Curry Chicken 55
Thai Coconut Curry Fish 48
Thai Papaya Salad 40
The Ultimate Arugula &
  Feta Salad 40
Tomato And Basil Baked Eggs With
  Artichokes 46
Trawberry Coconut Ice Cream 82
Tropical Berry Bliss Yogurt Bowl 78
Tropical Pineapple Kombucha 87
Tuna And Egg Salad With Olives 36
Tuna Salad Lettuce Wraps 51

Turkey And Vegetable Stew 33
Turkey Cobb Salad 39
Turmeric Coconut Energy Balls 82
Turmeric Hummus With Veggie
  Sticks 79
Turmeric Roasted Cauliflower 68
Turmeric-Tahini Dressing 75

V
Vegan Pancakes With Orange Zest
  And Chocolate Chips 44

W
Walnut Parsley Pesto 71
Walnuts And Dark
  Chocolate Bite 77
Watercress Salad 39
Watermelon Fermented Salsa 90
White Fish Stew 33

Z
Zesty Black Bean Soup 33
Zesty Chimichurri Sauce 72
Zucchini And Corn Salad 36
Zucchini Noodles With Pesto 69
Zucchini Pizza Bites 77
Zucchini Quinoa Frittata 59

Printed in Great Britain
by Amazon